# A Horse and Buggy Doctor
# Caught in the 21st Century

# A Horse and Buggy Doctor Caught in the 21st Century

By
**J.E. Block, M.D.**

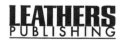

A division of Squire Publishers, Inc.
4500 College Blvd.
Leawood, KS 66211
1/888/888-7696

The opinions in this book are strictly those of the author and not necessarily those of any professional group. As a physician I do give medical advice, but on a specific individual basis. Therefore, nothing in this book should be construed as my medical opinion to the reader.

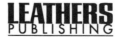

A division of Squire Publishers, Inc.
4500 College Blvd.
Leawood, KS 66211
1/888/888-7696

*This book is dedicated:*

*To my patients for the inspiration.*

*To my parents for the intellect.*

*And most of all, to my wife,
Brunhilde, and our eight children
for their sacrifices to allow me to
be the doctor I am today.*

# The Hippocratic Oath

*I swear by Apollo the physician, by Aesculapius, Hygeia, and Panacea, and I take to witness all the gods, all the goddesses, to keep according to my ability and my judgment the following oath:*

*To consider dear to me as my parents him who taught me this art; to live in common with him and if necessary to share my goods with him; to look upon his children as my own brothers, to teach them this art if they so desire without fee or written promise; to impart to my sons and the sons of the master who taught me and the disciples who have enrolled themselves and have agreed to the rules of the profession, but to these alone, the precepts and the instruction. I will prescribe regimen for the good of my patients according to my ability and my judgment and never do harm to anyone. To please no one will I prescribe a deadly drug, nor give advice which may cause his death. Nor will I give a woman a pessary to procure abortion. But I will preserve the purity of my life and my art. I will not cut for stone, even for patients in whom the disease is manifest; I will leave this operation to be performed by practitioners (specialists in this art). In every house where I come I will enter only for the good of my patients, keeping myself far from all intentional ill-doing and all seduction, and especially from the pleasures of love with women or with men, be they free or slaves. All that may come to my knowledge in the exercise of my profession or outside of my profession or in daily commerce with men, which ought not to be spread abroad, I will keep secret and will never reveal. If I keep this oath faithfully, may I enjoy my life and practice my art, respected by all men and in all times; but if I swerve from it or violate it, may the reverse be my lot.*

See new Oath, page 310.

# TABLE OF CONTENTS

## TABLES AND FIGURES

# ONE

# A Tattered Tale

## An Imperfect Medical System

An abundant life starts with pure internal and external environments. The discrete aggregation of mind, body and spirit allows our individual genetic endowments to produce, as God intended, an integrally happy human being, assuming appropriate pre and post natal care. Added to these influences is the ability to communicate internally by listening to our bodies, as well as externally by listening to our environment. A connection to a higher power, sincere companionship and a vital relationship with one's significant other are also key ingredients of life's recipe. Furthermore, volunteering to help folks, not taking ourselves too seriously, and knowing life is to be enjoyed, not endured, allow true expression of one's health. Health, therefore, encompasses much more than absence of illness.

In his 1988 *Doctors: The Biography of Medicine,* the famous historian and surgeon Sherwin B. Newland states that medical advances in the past twenty-five hundred years have come not from a steady continuum of progress, but from quantum leaps in knowledge and practice. Why then, despite the tremendous advances we have made scientifically, are we still, as a profession, third-rate physicians practicing fourth-rate medicine? It is not, I suggest, because of our selfishness, but because of traditional medical mindset. Most physicians have a blindness to many scientific studies that should confirm rather than refute medical theory. This response might be appropriate in other scientific endeavors, but medicine is an art based on scientific principles. Thus, research should verify hypotheses, confirm theories and document presumptive truths. However, because of our cultural biases and emotional prejudices, the evolution of medicine has been stuck in a quagmire of half-truths and pseudo-facts that sometimes borders on junk science. So, what we surmise as a medical fact today may well be false tomorrow. Over the past four decades as a physician I have seen this repeatedly. Medical knowledge is doubling every five years; we live in a forest of medical information, not knowing the true nature of the trees.

The relationship of estrogen and breast cancer is an example of this uncomfortable evolution. Prior to 1950 they were not related. In the late sixties, some literature suggested that giving estrogen to a woman post menopause might cause cancer. In the eighties there was proof in the literature that it actually caused cancer. By the early 'nineties, however, estrogen did not cause cancer of the breast but would accelerate its growth in women who already had the cancer. In 2000, we are giving estrogen to certain women with breast cancer! In the *New England Journal of Medicine* (Jan. 25, 2001: 276) the relationship between estrogen and breast cancer was finally revealed.

What, then, is a person to believe? While scientific breakthroughs in medicine uncover pieces of the puzzle, most conclude that still more research is needed to confirm the data and fit the pieces together. Medical knowledge is always in a state of flux. However, we live in today's world based on yesterday's facts, not tomorrow's assumptions. Thus, thousands of years of human experience should not be dismissed in favor of so-called modern scientific research. Both contribute to understanding health, and in the future the true relationship of hormones and cancer will be discovered.

The evolution of our medical perspective on tobacco in health demonstrates this conjunctive understanding. We have known intuitively for over a hundred years that smoking is bad for us. Still, tobacco companies tried to seduce us into thinking that it was not harmful. For instance, according to a 1951 advertisement in *Life* magazine (see page 3),

## Fig. 1-I
## In 1951, *Life Magazine* Advertised Camel Cigarettes as Being the Doctors' Choice

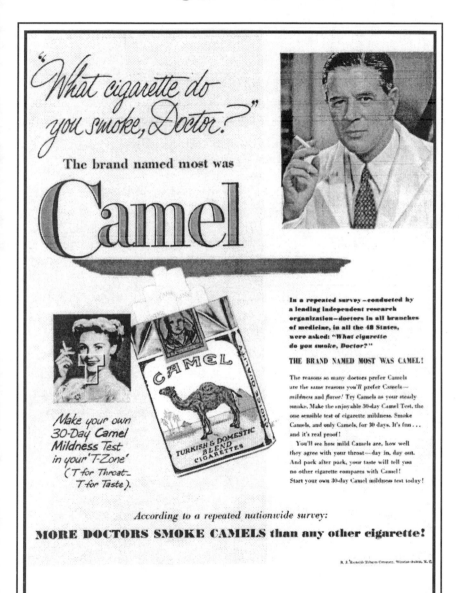

most doctors advised smoking, with over eighty-five percent smoking themselves. Today more than eighty-five percent do not smoke, much less advise it. It was not until 1964, though, that scientific research *proved* that smoking causes illnesses, and only now are the tobacco companies successfully being sued for injury in several states. The harmfulness of smoking is a medical truth that will never change.

Do we, then, need a hundred double blind studies costing billions of dollars to prove what your grandmother knew through common sense? The answer to this is both yes and no. At times, what we have believed to be true for a hundred years suddenly turns out to be false. For example, malaria is not caused by breathing bad air but, as Dr. Walter Read proved, by the bite of an infected mosquito. This kind of discovery is now popularized as evidence-based medicine. It reminds us to have open minds and to lift the iron curtain around the establishment who feel that if they did not learn it in medical school and if it is not published in several peer review medical journals, it is not so. Evidence-based medicine, however, must be understood in its current context: today most of us realize that what is published is either economically driven by pharmaceutical companies or is dictated by medical politics. Despite what mainstream medicine supports, what has not been proven scientifically is not necessarily disproved and can be useful in medical practice.

In this new millennium we should strive to increase the quality as well as the quantity of our lives. What good is a long life if one does not live well? At any age, we should be physically and mentally as young as possible. It is not important how old we are, but how we are when we are old. An old German saying states, *Alle Wuensche werden klein, gegen den — gesund zu sein,* "a healthy person has many desires, the sick individual has but one — to be healthy." Having a healthy life takes lots of work, good genes, faith, and a pinch of luck. Many of us believe that, like a broken piece of machinery, our bodies can be fixed as good as new. This is not so if we become injured or ill! With every illness, every disease, every trauma, a small but permanent disability remains. Thus, we must learn how to take better care of ourselves today so there will be minimal disability tomorrow. Of course, this is a truism, but how do we bring it to fruition in our own lives? Do we believe our doctor, the new health magazine, grandma or ourselves? Ultimately, being informed and assertive in our health care will give us the best chance for a healthier future. Hopefully, the rest of this book will give insight to this.

## An Ounce of Prevention

Ben Franklin had it right. It is certainly better to prevent disease than to simply treat disease. The former is referred to as prophylactic or preventative medicine, and the latter is known as crisis medicine. Most physicians (M.D.'s and D.O.'s), practice crisis medicine such as treating trauma (e.g., heart attack), infection (e.g., appendicitis) and sudden affliction to an organ (e.g., ulcer). The concept that many illnesses are a product of modern living on a planet different from that of our ancestors is paramount. The illnesses that occur because of this different environment are referred to as degenerative diseases. They include arthritis, arteriosclerosis, Alzheimer's disease, chronic fatigue syndrome, poor vision, and even aging.

Yes, aging, at least prematurely, is considered a disease by some. Genetically, we are destined to live 120-140 years; but, because of three factors — our environment, a decrease of glandular secretion (hormones), and faulty genes (those that decrease immunity or produce organ abnormalities) — we do not live to our life expectancy. As the genome project nears its end, we find that our genes are indeed malleable. One's life can vary depending on which gene is stimulated and which is suppressed by the environment. With the advent of genetic engineering we can begin life as perfect humans. Prenatal care will ensure that the untainted embryo will be programmed to be a healthy baby, and subsequently, a wholesome, mature person. Then the combination of crisis intervention and prevention will allow us not only to reach our full quality of life, but to stay in our prime for at least a century.

## Never Too Old

All that is needed for preservation of a species is for an organism to survive long enough to produce and nurture an offspring sufficiently to become free-living. In the case of humans this occurs when the mother has nourished, protected and taught her child how to make it alone in the world. The father often helps to nourish, protect and teach, although his primary biological purpose is to fertilize the egg. Subsequently, after producing two or more offspring, the parents are no longer needed for the maintenance of that species. After a given time, first the ovaries, then the other glandular secretions gradually decrease in the woman. The male maintains his testicular secretions (testosterone) almost all his life, but the secretions from the other glands similar to the female's dwindle.

Thanks to research, we can now replace or enhance almost all of these glandular fluids, or hormones. Thus, we do not have to succumb to the unnatural state of diminishing glandular function and disability. As a result, parents, grandparents and other adults work with children not only until they grow up to live alone, but can also continue the education, protection and nourishment until they're fully integrated into society. It is a delight to be a parent, a bigger joy to be a grandparent, and a jubilation to be a great-grandparent. Today, being a great-great-grandparent is the exception; tomorrow it will be the rule. After our reproductive years, humanity can continue to contribute to civilization in many other beneficial ways. Thus, the endeavors of people from maturity to death a century later will contribute to technical science, cultural discoveries, and to enhancing the lives of all humankind, both present and future. Although society has generally put older folks out to pasture, this is also changing. In the computer era, we will not be forced to retire just because of age, our community, and our current income tax structure.

We could be physically, mentally, and economically productive for as long as we desire.

## The World has Changed

A balanced union of the three pinnacles of mind, body and spirit will allow human beings to achieve their full destiny. The spirit, be it the Holy Spirit or a natural life force, must exist for us to exist. I do believe in a Divine Creator, but as a scientist, I also believe in evolution — not the classic Darwinian model, but a form of long term incremental development. Man has evolved over the last four hundred thousand years. Since research has disclosed that it takes at least twenty thousand years to produce a new species, we are still, metabolically, Paleolithic (cave men). As hunter-gatherers, our ancestors could, perhaps, have survived to one hundred twenty years if not for crisis illnesses and hazardous environmental conditions like inadequate food, shelter, and sanitation, as well as the presence of enemies. While our ability to treat and control these circumstances has improved, other hazards have evolved with modern society.

High density carbohydrates such as sugar, starches and alcohol are products of humanity's mental rather than physical evolution. Grains did not exist as a reliable food source until the last twelve thousand years. The great majority of us, then, are still not genetically adapted to eating high density carbohydrates like the starches and sugars engineered from grains, or alcohol fermented from plants. To add insult to injury, the minerals we need to stay at our metabolic best have diminished through the depletion of our soil over the centuries. Magnesium, for example, is a plant and animal mineral and an essential component of chlorophyll, a necessary catalyst for plant growth. Our magnesium intake is only a fraction of what it should be; in fact, almost forty percent of us are magnesium deficient when we reach the ripe age of twenty! The replacement of this important mineral is now known to "cure" hypertension, high cholesterol, diabetes, osteoporosis, muscle cramps, arthritis and heart disease. Similarly, minerals such as zinc, copper, iron, calcium, chromium, and selenium were abundant in the diet of our hunter-gatherer ancestors, but are not today. To make matters worse, our water has been "purified" to such an extent that the trace and rare minerals naturally included are now excluded.

If the deprivation of minerals is not enough to cause our modern-day diseases, the presence of toxins in our environment exacerbates our current less than ideal biochemistry. They can include chlorine in our water, pesticides in our food, hydrocarbons in our dry-cleaned clothes, radiation and electromagnetic waves to which we are exposed, noxious chemicals we apply to our bodies, and pollutants in the air. Furthermore, we now insulate our houses so much better for energy conservation than we did fifty years ago that we have tripled the concentration of some of these harmful compounds to which we are exposed.

## Faith as a Healer

Over twelve hundred research studies and reports indicate that spirituality and religion are extremely important determinants to health. In his book, *A Century of Research Reviewed,* Harold Koenig, M.D., includes an extensive discussion of the healing power of faith. For instance, in double-blind studies, bypass surgery patients who had no idea they were being prayed for did much better than a similar group for which there were no prayers. The prayers came from various denominations hundreds of miles away.

The healing power of faith is based not only on such mysterious components, but also on easily overlooked psychological principles. The physical and spiritual support of a temple, church, or mosque, for example, can help relieve a patient's sense of isolation and consuming obsession with his or her problems, thereby improving mental health and adaptation to disability. This, in turn, plays a large role in stress relief. The scientific relationship of stress and the immune system will be discussed in greater detail in Chapter Four. In this context of faith and healing, let us for now, suffice it to say that cytokines, natural inflammatory chemicals involved in many disease processes, that causes damage to our tissues, is significantly lower in patients who attended religious services compared to those who did not.

The lifestyle or behavior codes of many systems of faith also encourage good health. Negative health behaviors such as smoking and alcohol consumption are often tempered or prohibited. Moderation in personal and professional affairs, as well as in duty and pleasure, is widely advocated. Even for the generally healthy, religious activities are associated with a six- to ten-year longer survival than those who practice no religion, according to Dr. D. Oman in his in 1998 article in the *American Journal of Public Health.* Considering its spiritual, psychological, scientific, and common-sensical influence, it is no wonder that organized religion has grown by ten percent annually in America and is statistically correlated with a longer lifespan.

**The Waves of Energy**

Electromagnetic waves permeate the universe as well as our bodies and, therefore, do influence our health. Other bioenergetic systems such as the meridian concept used by acupuncturists and electro-conductive analysis are documented but poorly understood in terms of anatomy and biochemistry. In spite of our incomplete understanding, we know that, depending on the wavelengths, energy is transmitted from the invisible to the visible. Even the Bible commands, "Let there be light," but we do not get enough, nor the right kind. For eons humans bathed in light by day and hid in darkness by night. Civilization, however, has changed all this. We use artificial light at night and are deprived of the proper type of light during the day. The artificial light used in our homes, schools and workplaces is not full spectrum and therefore not nearly as good for our bodies as the sunlight we need. It is well known that SAD (Seasonal Affective Disorder) is caused by not getting enough outside light in the winter. Moreover, it has been found that the use of full spectrum light during the day is a successful treatment for some depressive disorders. Sleep disorders, daytime fatigue, and concentration are also improved by using such a light one hour before starting our day. Sleeping in a very dark, quiet room helps as well. At a lecture I attended a blind German professor exclaimed, "Even a blind person needs light to feel good." This entrainment of the circadian rhythm by melatonin in blind people has been documented by Dr. Robert Sach, et al, in the *New England Journal of Medicine* in October 12, 2000.

The skin produces vitamin D in response to sunlight. Sweat contains a pre-vitamin D form of cholesterol which is converted to the active vitamin D. This is used to create strong bones in the young and to prevent osteoporosis in the old. Certain spectrums of light (colors) change neuropeptides in the brain which not only elevate one's mood, but also heal. Various colors are used to treat maladies such as headaches, gastrointestinal problems, and congestion. Light exerts some of its effects through regulating the hormone, melatonin, produced in the pituitary gland. Melatonin helps us harmonize with changes in the environment, especially daily and seasonal transitions of sunlight.

Since the advent of artificial light civilization has been sleep deprived. In our working society sleeping too much is almost considered a sin. The proper amount of sleep, however, is crucial — for adults as well as children. Beginning in our teens we drastically cut down the hours of sleep that we get. Adults need at least eight hours of sleep. Insufficient sleep affects our mental and physiological functions. Insulin tolerance and immune responses, for instance, are markedly altered according to how much we sleep.

Accounting for and adjusting our "daily dose" of light waves is relatively easy and accessible. Electromagnetic waves are more pervasive but harder to keep track of. It is more than a theory that the magnetic field of the earth has been changing significantly over time. Our current understanding of electromagnetic fields implies wide potential health applications. A biomagnet based on rare earth minerals is coming on the market. This magnet is fifty times stronger than those usually available. Nonetheless, magnets have been applied for over three millennia in China and have been used for many medical ailments in most civilizations of the world. Arthur Philpot, M.D., of Oklahoma, has advanced research in biomagnetics considerably. Magnets do manipulate the bioelectric field of our tissues. Metaphorically, they restore the tissues to a proper "healing attitude." Magnets also decrease pain by aligning the atoms and the molecules in pain receptors in our ligaments. Some magnetic treatments restore the body to a normal state which is referred to as homeostasis, or a proper equilibrium of intrinsic micro-electrical forces.

In other words, magnets recharge the "human battery." For example, MDS (Magnetic Deficiency Syndrome) causes a gradual malfunctioning of various glands. Certain magnets referred to as "wafer magnets" (which can be obtained at health food stores) are placed on the sternum directly above the aorta, through which all the blood circulates. The magnetized blood then flows through and restores all our tissue, resulting in the return of health. More specific applications are also used. For dizziness, the magnet is placed on the back of the neck. When pain exists, it is placed near that area. (Pregnant women, however, should not use the magnet on the abdomen.) For acid indigestion, a magnet on top of the stomach works well. For quick relief of a headache, the magnet is placed over the area of the head which hurts the most, but with some headaches such as migraines, the magnet is often more effective in the upper area of the back and neck. It can even be used with toothaches. Magnetic therapy seems to work better if one takes calcium and magnesium supplements with it. Norman Schille, M.D., of the Springfield, Missouri Pain Clinic, has also experimented with magnets for depression. He puts one above the bridge of the nose and another on the small lump normally found in the middle of the skull on the back of the head. This is used for one hour each morning along with a bright, full spectrum light. According to his research, the depression resolves in less than two weeks! Bioenergy and electrodynamics are as much a part of healing as are the medicines that doctors prescribe.

## Captain of the Team

Most physicians go into medicine for the proper humanitarian reasons, to help people. To be a tattle tale, though, I must admit that many of us emerge from medical training with a different spin on life. Most doctors end up overly self-interested, looking for both ego and economic fulfillment. Rare individuals retain their calling and remain compassionate healers. How, then, does a patient find a physician who thinks with his mind and feels with his heart? We need someone who is kind, who has time to listen, and who is seasoned, but not too young nor too old. He or she should be accessible and, most importantly, know the mind-body interaction. He or she should be open-minded enough to respect our opinions on both conventional and non-conventional therapies. I am referring to a primary care doctor who, if he is good, knows what they know and, more significantly, knows what they do not know. And if he or she does not know, he or she will find someone for us who does!

Frequently though, there is a gap between what we expect as a patient and what we get. In these days of managed care, we are often assigned a doctor rather than being able to choose one. If you are medically knowledgeable, and after reading this book you should be, I recommend interviewing your prospective physician. Offer to pay for his or her time. In addition to the usual questions about fees and insurance coverage, ask how he or she feels about disease prevention, nutrition and natural remedies. You should be the captain of your medical team, and your physician the coach. Make sure the staff is courteous, helpful and treats you like an individual, not like another patient in need of medical help. The yellow pages, county medical society secretaries, and hospitals have lists of primary care physicians. They are referenced as family practitioners, general practitioners or general internists. However, asking friends or family about their doctors seems to work better. With the upcoming legislation even managed care patients can pick an appropriate physician of their choice, if they are insistent.

## My Tale

The desire to become a physician is multifaceted, based simultaneously on money, prestige, science, adulation, a good life, the ability to help humanity, and voyeurism. Yes, in a study several years ago, a fair number of prospective doctors volunteered that seeing a nude body was one of the unvoiced reasons to be a physician. Thus, in the spirit of fairness, I'll do a little disrobing of my own; the following is my case history, offered for your scrutiny.

My family moved from Philadelphia, Pennsylvania, to Atlantic City, New Jersey, when I was four years old. I was the product of a manic-depressive mother and a hypochondriacal father. This cross-fertilized my soul to go into a healing profession. Like many families in those days, we were poor but I didn't know it.

In the 1940s, eighty-five percent of physicians were general practitioners with the rest being specialists. I knew little of specialists outside of a surgeon who did a right-sided hernia repair on me at age five and another who did the left when I was fourteen. Instead, I wanted to be like the doctor who came to my house when I was very ill. He gave me a shot and the next day I was better. Of course, I probably had a virus and the injection of penicillin did not contribute to my improvement. This was before the time of antibiotic resistant bacteria brought on by such injudicial use of these drugs.

Unfortunately, my performance in school provided little support for my desire. Being a poor student, I floundered through grade school. Despite being held back in the fifth grade, I still did poorly for the next six grades. I probably had Attention Deficient Hyperactivity Disorder (ADHD), but that syndrome wasn't known then and my parents and teachers wrote me off as a bad boy. And, indeed, I lived up to the designation, getting into trouble at school, after school, at home or anywhere I spent my time. I not only drove my parents and teachers to distraction, but also ended up in the police station more than once.

My peer group all vowed to become professionals to improve their socio-economic status, and I went along with the crowd. Thanks to a good friend whom I met during my first year in high school whose father was a physician, I opted for that profession. Based on my miserable high school grades, my guidance counselor had other thoughts. The lack of junior colleges and the G.I. bill for returning Korean Conflict veterans made it hard for a poor student to matriculate in a halfway decent pre-medical school. To get into college in the fifties, I had to survive the college boards, which, like SATs and ACTs, were the pre-admission tests of that era.

I took a book out of the library to help prepare my mathematic and verbal skills for the "big test." I managed to memorize ten thousand big words, and I was already good at reading because when I did go to class I usually read a book rather than paid attention. Perhaps I was lucky, for when the results came back I'd scored in the top one percent of the country in the verbal half of the test. The math, which I mainly flunked in school, was more worrisome. I could not add, subtract, divide or multiply well, but in spacial math I excelled. On a geometry test, for instance, I once got the highest grade in the class. Of course, I was accused of cheating by looking at my neighbor's paper, but was soon acquitted when I explained that if I cheated, I could not get a better grade than he did. Fortunately, the math part of the college boards was practically designed for me. It consisted of mazes through which to find the right path, series of numbers in which I had to pick those that didn't belong, and various questions that required common sense rather than fundamental math skills. When my math score was returned, I landed in the top two percent of the country.

My high board results allowed me to apply at various colleges for interviews. Still, many would not grant me one because of my abysmal grades and worse recommendations from my teachers. One college finally did, and later accepted me, provisionally, on the condition that I do well. Muhlenberg College in Allentown, Pennsylvania, had, reputedly, a good pre-medical program; one hundred percent of the students would get accepted into medical school — because those who did not make excellent grades were simply kicked out of the program. Consequently, I will never forget my first college test, which was in Ancient History. I received a thirty-two! I thought that I would soon be history.

Chuck Kahn, my college roommate, the influential friend I mentioned earlier whose father was a physician, came to my rescue. Having already attended a year at the University of Pennsylvania, he knew how to study, imparted in painful detail by his father. Chuck taught me how to study — and study I did, eight to twelve hours a day, in addition to attending classes and trying to earn a living. Thankfully, this focus on productivity and frugality was already, for better or worse, familiar to me. I had worked since I was seven years old, first selling newspapers on street corners and in the local taverns. As I grew older, I had various, and often simultaneous, jobs as an entrepreneur, working my way through grade and high school. This experience helped me master school just in time; for at age twenty I married a girl of sixteen. By my senior year (before the advent of birth control pills) I had my first daughter — so I had to work harder than ever to make enough money to support my new family and a college education. By the time I applied to medical school I was tenth in my college class of over four hundred and was easily accepted at Seton Hall College of Medicine, which was then the only medical school in New Jersey. It is now called New Jersey College of Medicine.

Like most medical schools, Seton Hall required two years of basic science. This included anatomy, physiology, biochemistry and a smattering of clinical subjects such as laboratory medicine and physical diagnosis. After the two years of basic science, I did my clinical rotation in pediatrics, OB-GYN, surgery, and internal medicine. With each rotation I went through, I changed my mind in favor of becoming that kind of doctor. I eventually had to settle on one and chose internal medicine. Soon I was off to California for my internship and residency at University of Southern California and later a UCLA hospital. After my internship, I longed so much to be in practice that I went into general practice for two years, and it did my heart good. Like in medical school, I could be all those specialists — pediatrician, obstetrician, and surgeon — at once. It was wonderful. I delivered over two hundred babies in my training! But it was the obstetrics that took me out of general practice in 1966 and back to specializing only in internal medicine. A very difficult delivery was the deciding point. The mother was in labor for over thirty-six hours, and the baby barely breathed at first. That was the last baby I delivered. Several years later, I saw the child and mother and, thank God, both were fine. I knew that if I had had a residency in OB-GYN and delivered two thousand rather than two hundred babies I could, perhaps, have done a better job and not jeopardized the life of that child.

After my residency I taught full-time for a year at UCLA—Harbor General Hospital, and then moved to the Midwest to practice and teach part-time at several medical schools. In 1980, I left practice and taught full-time at the University of Missouri in Kansas City. Part of my responsibility as a teacher at the medical school was to provide continuing medical education to practicing physicians, so I went to distant communities three or four times a month to lecture on various medical subjects. In 1984, I flew to a small town at the edge of the state to talk about high blood pressure. I am not sure if it was the ambiance of this rural cowboy town or too much red wine at dinner before my talk, but I stated boldly that if I were ever to go into practice again, it would be in a community just like this one. Little did I know that a physician in the audience not only picked up the nuances of the current diagnosis and treatment for high blood pressure, but also my cowboy assertion. Several days later, I received a phone call from that doctor explaining that he was in the hospital with what could be terminal cancer. He confessed that in twenty minutes he would undergo surgery and that he was not confident of surviving. He wanted to pass me the torch he lit twenty years earlier. This doctor felt that I was one of the few physicians who could take over his practice properly and care for his patients — who, incidentally, were his friends.

Needless to say, I was flattered, and the physician in me agreed on the spot to help this poor human being. That way he could have at least some peace while going through his current ordeal. I knew both my wife and the medical school would protest; the former because we had just finished restoring a house which was to be placed on the National Historic Registry, and the latter because I was the chief of medicine at the main satellite teaching hospital of the University, and no one was waiting in the wings to replace me. Refusing to take no for an answer from my wife and indicating to the medical school that they would have to sue me for breach of contract, I packed my medical belongings and, within a month, was in the rural town practicing medicine — initially without my wife. The physician who invited me to take over his practice did come out of surgery but never practiced again and, within a year, succumbed to his malignancy.

So here I was, in a small town that I had dreamed about ever so long, ready to be a real practicing doctor. Shortly after my move, my wife decided that I had not taken leave of my senses, and since this was what I really wanted to do with my life, she joined me. I fulfilled some of my obligations to the medical school by flying the four hundred miles once or twice a week to teach until they found someone else. In those days I was a private pilot — until I crashed and totaled my plane; but that is another story.

During my first month in this rural area one of my colleagues handed me a book called *The Horse and Buggy Doctor* by Arthur E. Hetzler. I savored every word of it and said to myself, "When I grow up, I want to be just like him." Born in 1869, Dr. Hetzler began his medical career as a true pioneer doctor. Initially without a hospital, he did it all, operating many times on a kitchen table with primitive instruments after a twenty-hour buggy ride to some wilderness farm. Still, his success rate rivaled that of our modern facilities. His pragmatic wisdom in dealing with the human animal and our subtleties, ambiguities, and eccentricities which color both disease and non-disease alike, should be emulated by all physicians. He reminded me once again of the art of medicine: one hundred years ago it was based on a lot less science than it is today. Dr. Hetzler eventually built his own clinic and hospital in Halstead, Kansas, which, in the 1950s, was considered the Mayo Clinic of the lower Midwest. Writing several scientific books and publishing medical articles firmly established him as my practitioner hero of yesteryear. Similarly, in my earlier years William Osler (Chapter Nine) was my academic demigod.

With my medical background and Dr. Hetzler's influence, I, too, initiated a rural practice to lessen human suffering and stop premature death. Like he, I alienated many of my colleagues and battled with my local hospital. My frustration with hospitals is both fundamental and incidental. Generally, there are too many hospitals, and they are overly competitive. Each hospital is composed of two parts, the physical plant and its philosophy. The latter is determined by the administration and several of the influential medical staff who may or may not be good physicians. This faction conducts the business of the hospital, often with a bloated sense of economic and professional self-interest. In our rural area it was malevolent, to say the least. As I was unwilling to tolerate such blatant disregard for patient welfare, I went from chief of staff to the bottom of the graph of our local hospital and was exiled later.

Nonetheless, or more likely, as a result, I have encompassed more spheres of medicine with more healing possibilities than most of my colleagues who have held themselves back in the orthodox, allopathic mode. Allopathic medicine need not be exclusive; it is preserved by our Western (scientific) cultural biases. The allopathic can proceed to naturopathic, heliopractic, chiropractic and other non-traditional healing philosophies that are just now being explored in our medical schools.

Fortunately or unfortunately, my practice continued to grow. Hopefully, there will be an end to it. With five clinicians, thirty employees, and a large physical plant, we bring to our community a formidable medical group that will truly be, not just on the cutting edge of the new medicine, but a team that makes its decisions in practice with the heart as well as the mind. The Patch Adams in me will always make me stand out from the crowd as he has, for better or for worse. Hopefully, it will be for the better, not for my sake, but for the sake of my patients, their loved ones, and the future of medicine.

## An Internist

An internist is a specialist in diagnosing and healing the internal organs such as the heart, lung, kidney and brain. The sub-specialists of internal medicine are the cardiologist, the pulmonologist, the nephrologist and the neurologist. They know the diseased organ, but not the patient. The general internist is usually a primary care doctor whose job is to put all of the pieces of the patient puzzle together to get a clear picture of the total medical and human situation. He or she then acts as a guide in helping the patient choose the correct path.

General internists, then, diagnose diseases, and with these diagnoses, we treat. This combination is based on medical judgment, not on a practice guide handed out by an HMO. It is based on the pathophysiology (what and why things have gone wrong) of the individual. This medical judgment develops in medical school, from current text books and medical journals, and most of all, through our practical experience. Continuing medical education lectures, both flawed and ideal, published clinical trials and what we have observed from our colleagues' patients influence how we diagnose and treat. Involving the patient in the decision is most important. I now know that all patients are not created equal and the same therapeutic regime that works for one may not for another. Patients are not guinea pigs, but everything in medicine is a therapeutic trial. This is the individualism of medicine, which I will discuss in greater detail in Chapter Two.

## A Shift in Medical Thinking

It is not who is right, but what is right that counts. Alternative medicine is being rediscovered and slowly shifting the medical paradigm; what used to be considered non-scientific bunk, some physicians now think is the correct method of healing a patient. One of the main reasons physicians are hesitant to use alternative medicine is the lack of scientific proof or explanation of its effectiveness. Conventionally trained allopathic physicians evaluate alternative medicine through the biomechanical model, and not through the general systems theory, which is more plausible to the variations of the human organism. Therefore, Chinese, Ayurvedic, Herbal, Electromagnetic medicine, etc., could, but do not, make sense to physicians who have had orthodox medical training. There are several important differences between the biomechanical model we learned in medical school, and the general systems hypothesis, espoused by alternative physicians. The general systems theory considers quantum physics which can explain sudden, unexpected changes in a person's health. It sees an individual as a total organism rather than a biological machine. The individual strives to maintain stability through homeostasis, keeping all parts of the body in balance. Thus, a sudden perturbation may be interpreted by the organism as a crisis in which the body releases potentially noxious chemicals into the blood stream. The individual then identifies the disturbance and influences it. If, for a simple example, we are cold, we shiver. When such attempts to harmonize our internal and external circumstances fail, disease is the result!

As the changing of medical paradigms suggests, in the long run society is frugal; that is, what is not practical has generally been thrown out over millennia. We have scientifically and philosophically revised medicine again and again. In particular, Oriental and other older forms of medicine long ago rid themselves of what did not work; and what has survived does work. Although the yin-yang proposition holds little validity to most Western physicians, and the meridian concept with *Chi* may be considered heretical by mainstream doctors, both should have a place in modern medicine. There is a definite need for these types of diagnoses and treatments. In Oriental and Ayurvedic medicine feeling the pulse, inspecting the tongue, and somehow sensing what sickness the patient has are methods used to diagnose and treat the patient. Some diseases with which modern medicine has a poor track record, such as chronic fatigue syndrome, fibromyalgia, and irritable bowel, may be better diagnosed and treated by these other disciplines.

If a physician cannot account for the underlying explanation of an illness, based on the scientific reasoning learned from allopathic medicine, he or she may relegate the patient's problem to the head and not to the body. But if a doctor can otherwise intuit what is going on, he or she is not arbitrarily assigning a cause and can greatly help a patient even though it cannot be documented on the patient's conventional medical chart. A physician is not a magician. Diagnosis and treatment is a logic based on relativity such as was claimed by Einstein rather than on the older static mechanical physics embraced centuries earlier by Newton. Of course, in today's science both Newton and Einstein are correct and the world accepts both. So, why can't this happen with orthodox medicine and non-conventional medical concepts? A holistic approach is the only way to treat some disease states. Why not present the best of both possible worlds to an individual who may need one or the other or, possibly, a combination of these philosophies? The following chapters will expand on this more realistic approach to health.

## Mind Over Matter

A good doctor endeavors to help the body repair itself, to awaken the healer within. Thus, we try to approach a patient from several different directions to see what is the most beneficial. This will lead the patient down the correct track toward regained health, preserved wholeness, and a satisfying and salubrious life. At any given time the total health of a patient is determined by a series of factors, the most important of which is genetics.

In the past, we have thought of genetics as a fixed determinant. Certainly hair color, skin color, eye color, and height are not easily changed without the help of hair dye, UV light, tinted contact lenses, and growth hormone. We are discovering, however, that much of the genetic code is malleable. Even at the molecular level we are finding that the environment determines genetic expression. Under certain external conditions the biochemistry of a given piece of the genetic code is stimulated, but under different circumstances another part of the genetic code is activated. In other words, the same set of genes will manifest different characteristics in response to the environment.

Therefore, almost ironically, our environment determines whether or not we will get an inherited disease like coronary artery disease, breast cancer, prostrate cancer or diabetes. For after genetics, the second basic component of the body's structure is the actual building blocks used to create the individual: food, drink, and air provide the molecules of which we are composed. Certainly, if one gives the body faulty building materials or fills it with toxins that interfere with its ideal structure, the body will be weakened and vulnerable.

This molecular matter is given specific instructions by certain chemicals or neuropeptides, sometimes termed neurotransmitters. This area of medicine, which I'll refer to as *Psychoneuroimmunology,* suggests that neuropeptides produced in the brain and other sites have a profound effect on every part of the body via the receptors responding to these neurotransmitters. Even thinking creates neuropeptides. Thus, this is truly mind over matter. The condition of illness or health certainly is in the patient's head, but is activated at distant locations through these neuropeptides and their receptors in various tissues. This dynamic represents a dialogue of sorts; the mind tells the tissues and the tissues inform the mind.

What we think of as the meaning of our illness is also important. Past experiences and beliefs influence our historical neurochemistry, which creates a balance, or in cases of "dis-ease," a dysfunction. An individual recognizes the constellation of symptoms in reference to his or her experience. Thus, it is not just the number of doctor visits or the specific treatments that make us better, but our relationship to, or historical interpretation of the illness. Thus, I frequently ask a patient what he feels is the significance of his medical problem.

Even when we try to listen to our bodies, they do not always speak clearly. They really speak in metaphors, which require interpretation. People can, in fact, die of a broken heart; a mother can be a pain in the neck, and a job a pain in the ass! Certainly, these patients will complain of chest, neck and sacroiliac pain. This may be a reflection of life's stresses and imposed disability. The symptoms of an illness therefore do have meaning, both literally and figuratively.

Given this interpenetration of mind and matter, it's not what is scientifically proven, but what is proper for the patient that counts. Some illnesses, like trauma or heart attacks, are best treated by conventional orthodox medicines. Others, such as chronic pain syndrome, may best be treated by Chinese acupuncture, or other non-conventional medical philosophies. This is why I choose a holistic approach to treating a patient. I learned years ago that the average practitioner treats symptoms and a good doctor treats the disease, but the best physician treats the patient!

*"Treat people as though they were what they ought to be and you will help them become what they are capable of being."*
—*Goethe*

## Figure 1-II

### Weight Loss the Easy Way

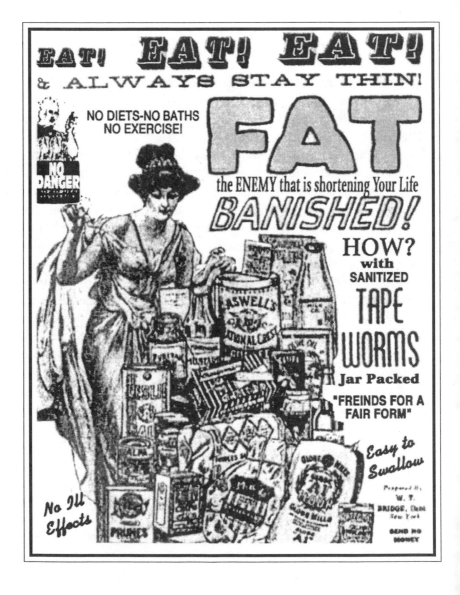

TWO

# The End of Medical Innocence

## Dissatisfaction

Dissatisfaction encourages people to change. This was true even in the mythological origins of medicine. Aesculapius, (also referred to as Asclepias and Asklepias), the son of Apollo, defied the gods and was struck down by Zeus for interfering with "divine' (often whimsical) order by relieving suffering and rescuing those stricken with death. His staff, on which the magical healing serpent ascends, is the emblem of our healing profession. In his 1996 article, "Asklepias: Ancient Hero of Medical Caring," published in *Archives of Internal Medicine*, J.E. Bradley, M.D., explains that Asklepias evokes the true heart of a physician, reminding us to have a personal bond with our patients and to make their individual welfare a prime consideration. For his compassion, skill, and dedication Aesculapius is mentioned in the Hippocratic Oath. He should not, however, be confused with Hippocrates, the true father of modern medicine in whose honor medical school graduates take this oath (see Page ii).

Like Aesculapius, many physicians today are dissatisfied with the imposed or unquestioningly accepted limitations on healing taught in orthodox medical schools and post-graduate curricula. Counting myself among the disenchanted, I was privileged to hear James Gordon, M.D., from Washington, D.C. speak to a group of health professionals in Ann Arbor, Michigan. Much of the following is from this talk and his book, *The Manifesto of the New Medicine*.

As conventional physicians, we have seen our patients drift off increasingly to other "healthcare providers," both those who are qualified and those who are not. In a recent study, fifty-four percent of patients saw alternative practitioners in the twelve months preceding a visit to their medical doctor and, more importantly, less than half told their physicians about the other forms of treatment. Patients are clearly dissatisfied, and so, for that matter, are physicians. A survey in 1998 found that thirty-six percent of doctors said they would not go into medicine again if they were given the opportunity. Fortunately, the remaining sixty-four percent, like I, would do so again and again. Indeed, many of my colleagues are dropping out of medicine not because the profession is too demanding, but because the standards of care have changed drastically. We no longer use thorough history-taking and physical examination for a clinical diagnosis. Instead, we make our diagnoses from expensive and frequently useless tests, the byproducts of technological advancement. Please do not misunderstand; I think technology enriches the health and welfare of all humankind. In our society, however, patients as well as doctors demand the latest tests, which frequently clarify nothing. Furthermore, the risks of many invasive testing procedures far outweigh the proposed benefits.

A problem with orthodox allopathic medicine can also obscure the focus of treatment. Often, the disease is treated rather than the patient who suffers with the disease. We were taught textbook cases of disease but seldom see such a classic patient because there are many variations of a sickness. A colleague once said to me, "Diseases can have as many faces as a patient pleases." What happens in one individual with a certain illness may be completely different than another. Some patients have no symptoms, while others have subclinical or non-specific ones, and depending on the environment and constitutional background, still another could die from the same disease process. We as physicians may inherently know such a range of affliction exists, but it seldom enters into our therapeutic thinking of patient care, making us less effective than we should be.

Until the first decade in the twentieth century physicians incorporated the best of all known medical philosophies, combining homeopathic, herbal, ancient as well as ultra-modern (e.g., electromagnetic) healing modalities in their practices. This was referred to as eclectic medicine. The problem with this heterogeneity was a lack of standards in both medical education and practice. Consequently, the Carnegie Foundation sponsored a commission headed by the well-known academic physician Abraham Flexner which published a report in 1910 that led to an almost instantaneous revision of the medical arts. Many of these methods were shown to be scientifically insupportable and thus were cast out. Doctors using these therapeutic techniques were branded as quacks and charlatans. In the tidal wave of this mindset, those healing therapies — many of which did have great value — have been slow to resurface. Now, even when scientific background accompanies their reemergence, these forms of eclectic medicine are still not accepted by most mainstream physicians

## The Law of Consequences

As I mentioned earlier, it is not who is right but what is right that counts. This statement is based in part on a natural law that operates in the universe called "The Law of Consequences:" every action will have a reaction, and for every act we perform there is a natural and appropriate consequence. What follows comes not from research, but from my heart. I feel sorry for many people I see in the news each day. The radio, television, and newspapers are filled with stories of those who either didn't know about the "Law of Consequences" or thought it would not catch up with them when they committed immoral, unethical or illegal acts. Unfortunately, these folks failed to realize they were just sowing seeds that would sooner or later come up, exposing selfishness and corruption for all to see. Even if their malicious actions were never revealed, dark secrets take an even greater toll. For we can never escape from who we really are or the intimate consequences of our actions. When we commit a serious misdeed its malignancy stays with us as long as we live.

On the other hand, while all pernicious acts consume life, all just and compassionate ones nurture and renew it. In this sense, the law of consequences allows us to tell our own fortunes. When our actions are based on truth, honesty, and integrity, over time good things will come to us. This is not to say that bad things do not happen to good people. We all know they do. When we face hardship or injury we need not ask, "Why me?" but rather, "How will I respond?" If one has a good heart there are no mistakes, only lessons. We will learn and grow from our misfortune.

The earth can provide for our needs, but not our greed. Egocentrism teases us with immediate and tangible results, but altruism is more fulfilling and rewarding. A lot of good people fail to realize all the blessings they can receive from being of service to others. If we just look for ways to help other people, with the right attitude and the right motive, more good will come our way than we ever dreamed possible.

## An Antidote to Antibiotics

Health care consumers are voting with their wallets, choosing to spend more healthcare dollars on supplements and alternative medicine than on traditional care, even though it may be subsidized by third party carriers. This trend is admirable and hopefully will decrease some of the problems we are having with microbial resistance to the antibiotics on the market now, as well as those in the future. As practicing community physicians, we are accused of abusing rather than using antibiotics appropriately. Hence we are blamed for the increasing anti-microbial resistance that the modern world is experiencing. This incidental over-prescribing, however, represents only the tip of the iceberg.

A significant factor associated with bacterial resistance is increased antibiotic use in hospitals where these drugs are used empirically rather than after bacterial cultures and sensitivities to the drug are obtained. Instead of a narrow spectrum antibiotic for a specific bug, many hospitalists use a broad spectrum drug. Repeated antibiotic courses and prolonged hospitalizations compound the problem. Intensive-care unit ecology, the immunocompromised state of the patient, increased use of invasive devices and catheters, ineffective infection control procedures, and inter-hospital transfers of colonized patients should likewise be considered.

International travel has also been implicated, but the real culprit is animal husbandry and agricultural use. Annually, in the United States, approximately eight million kg of anti-microbial agents are used for animals and twenty-two thousand kg are used for fruit trees. The antibiotics used in agriculture and agrifood industries are numerous, including chlortetracycline, erythromycin, bacitracin, penicillin, streptomycin and lincomycin. Antibiotics engineered for animals and plants usually precede those used for humans and fight many of the same bacteria that infect humans. This allows the development of bacteria already resistant when the drug is finally approved for human use. Many veterinarian drugs such as sarafloxacin are very closely related to those used in humans like ciprofloxacin. Vancomycin resistance in our hospitals of staph and enterococci is already here. Thankfully, awareness is on the rise. On December 31, 2000, the FDA had requested two fluoroquinalone antibiotics by Bayer and Abbott Laboratories to be taken off the market.

Using herbal and complementary medicine techniques to boost a person's immune defense will decrease antibiotic usage, thereby limiting the emergence of resistant bacteria strains. The development of antiviral agents, which is coming at an incredible pace, will supplement this process. So I advise not taking an antibiotic for a minor infection which is more likely than not, viral. Children, perhaps at the parent's insistence, are given antibiotics for trivial reasons. While this is good for the pharmaceutical companies, it is bad for the patient and our planet.

# Table 2-I

## Alternative Therapies

Acupuncture
Applied Kinesiology
Aromatherapy
Ayurvedic Medicine
Biofeedback Training
Biological Dentistry
Bodywork
Botanical Medicine
Chelation Therapy
Chiropractic
Colon Therapy
Craniosacral Therapy
Detoxification Therapy
Diet Therapy
Electrical Therapy
Energy Medicine
Environmental Medicine
Enzyme Medicine
Fasting
Flower Remedies
Guided Imagery
Homeopathy
Iridology
Juice Therapy

Kinergetics
Light Therapy
Live Cell Therapy (Thymus)
Magnetic Field Therapy
Massage Therapy
Meditation
Mind/Body Medicine
Motion Therapy
Naturopathic Medicine
Neural Therapy
Neuro-Linguistic Programming
Nutritional Supplements
Orthomolecular Medicine
Osteopathy
Oxygen Therapy
Ozone Therapy
Qigong
Reconstructive Therapy
Reicke
Reflexology
Sound Therapy
Touch Therapy
Traditional Chinese Medicine
Yoga

The above is a partial list. Other healing treatments have been described, and there are several sub-categories of most of those listed.

## Definitions

Only now is the pendulum starting to swing from mainstream medicine to *Alternative Medicine*. Alternative means "other than." It includes everything that we medical students did not learn in school and what is not customarily practiced in our clinics and hospitals. Perhaps, in the last several years some of us may have been discovering what we did not in our formal studies. The good news is that recently some medical schools have added the alternative therapies (see Table 2-I, page 30) to their curriculums. Complementary Medicine, a British term, indicates those alternatives that can complement, or add to conventional medicine.

Holistic Medicine is a term that was first used in Western scientific literature in 1926 by Jan Christian Smuts, a South African biologist and statesman who wrote the book *Holism and Evolution*. The term comes from the Greek word, "holos," for whole. The concept is the whole is greater than the sum of its parts. This is true of any organism. On the other hand, Bacon and Descartes, famous philosophers in the 16th century, believed that to know an organism one must dissect and understand it in progressively smaller parts. Through this kind of analysis, they declared, we will know the truth of a living creature. Dr. Kurt Goldstine offered yet another thesis which was, perhaps, more germane: the organistic theory. He was a well-known psychiatrist who worked with men who had been brain damaged in World War I due to trauma. Goldstine found that contrary to some of the outstanding research done previously in brain localization and function of the body, most patients who had major portions of their brains shot away — parts that were supposedly responsible for particular actions — were still able to carry out those functions, demonstrating the brain's capacity to reorganize itself and the premise of holistic medicine. This notion began in 1922, but only a few biologists espoused it until the 1970s. The lay definition of holistic medicine today includes the entire field of various non-orthodox medical healing procedures such as acupuncture or magnetic therapy, as well as orthodox medicine. The holistic physician will use whatever it takes, conventional and eclectic, to heal the patient.

*Mind-Body Medicine* emphasizes the effects of the mind on the body and the body on the mind. The complete interaction of mind over body is well known, but the reverse is not. The discovery in the 1940s of neurotransmitters established that the body could indeed talk to the mind as much as the brain could communicate with the body. An all inclusive moniker might, in the German style of word grafting, be *psychoneuroimmunoendocrinology*. Research has revealed that the very same receptors and neurotransmitters, or peptides, are present in the cells of the brain, the endocrine system, peripheral nervous system, immune system, as well as all the organs of the body. This provides for ongoing feedback among virtually every system in every organ of the body. Mind-Body Medicine seeks to enter this conversation, and improve the level of discourse of the entire human being. The mind, then, does enhance both physical and psychological well-being. The same neurotransmitters also work in reverse, modulating, for better or worse, mood and mental functioning. We will discuss this relationship more in reference to Chronic Fatigue Syndrome and Fibromyalgia under "The F Word" in chapter Six.

*Integrative Medicine* technically has a different connotation than Holistic Medicine. It involves integrating different healing modalities and healing systems, including the essences of primitive, ancient, arcane, and technological healing paradigms that have not yet, or perhaps never will, become mainstream. Examples of primitive forms of healing are acupuncture and herbology, which date back to the cave man. Ayurvedic (continental Indian) and Chinese traditional medicine illustrate ancient forms of the healing arts that, indeed, worked. Homeopathy is considered an arcane form, while high-tech medicine includes natural and electromagnetic vibrational energy transference devices. Integrative Medicine also draws on chiropractic and various forms of mind-body healing such as meditation, hypnosis and the most practiced — religion. Healing by faith has existed for five millennia and will continue until the end of time. Accordingly, Integrative Medicine can also bridge the gap between conventional Western medicine and non-conventional healing. In 1997 the Capital University of Integrative Medicine was established in Washington, D.C. It is a two-year post graduate school for practitioners who already have a degree in a conventional curriculum. They can then continue another year to write a thesis and obtain a Ph.D. I am enrolled in that institution at the present.

## New and Improved

For the first time on this planet we have the opportunity and the inclination to integrate these many approaches. The breed that emerges from this manifold fertilization is *The New Medicine*. We now try to understand the healing arts that have been used in various cultures throughout time and incorporate them into our practices. Though these other disciplines are not new, bringing them together with Western science is. I also like the term, The New Medicine, because it never goes out of date; what is new is always evolving, and medicine should, too. Consider the transformation of what we now think of as modern medicine. More and more research for chronic illness concludes there are no "magic bullets," a term coined by the great physician, Paul Ehrlich. He found, in the late 1880s, a "cure" for syphilis: when physicians started using arsenic for the disease it was thought to be a godsend. But as the months and years rolled on some patients became fatally ill because of the treatment: the cure was worse than the disease. Thus the term, magic bullet. The concept has evolved, and some bullets, although not magic, do indeed help—like using antibiotics for bacterial infections. Still, these bullets start ricocheting, producing antibiotic-resistant bacteria. In some cases we are no better at treating certain infections than in Dr. Ehrlich's time. However, using the best of the old, the recent, and the forthcoming, the New Medicine can help our patients far more than the so-called standard or allopathic medicine alone.

The lack of individuality, partnership, and self-care in today's medical system also drive us toward a new medicine. One has to look no farther than the celebrated Patch Adams for the individual practice philosophy in physician-patient relationships. It is well documented that being light-hearted and happy uniquely improves our immune systems. Perhaps Norman Cousins was correct when he wrote his book, *Laughter Is the Best Medicine*. There are, understandably, peculiarities that bring those giving care and those seeking it together. Most patients who come to my practice do so because they want another approach that they feel will be more successful than what they have received. Frequently, they want a method that will help them feel better while another therapy takes hold, such as giving a potent anti-inflammatory for acute rheumatoid arthritis while waiting for a disease modifying agent to take effect. Another example is cancer patients undergoing radiation and chemotherapy. This may get rid of the cancer, but what about the poor patients? They are miserable, fatigued and without immunity. To this end, the famous cancer hospital in Houston, Texas, the MD Anderson, started a cancer fatigue clinic in 1998. Inevitably, patients come to the New Medicine for alternatives, and find the doctors actually spending time listening to them. This is what is visualized on TV, not just the old "Marcus Welby" approach, but also the recent Gideon's Crossing. A major factor in switching health care providers is that patients believe they will receive more attention from doctors who say they are holistic, alternative, complementary, or integrated because these practitioners will take more time and pay more attention to the other aspects of a patient's life.

Another major force driving this mild revolution is health maintenance organizations (HMOs). They are maintaining, but not enhancing people's health by preventing disease. Furthermore, the less time health professionals have for people under the guise of efficiency, the more the patients resent that system. Some HMOs are starting to allow alternative medicine. This results in more satisfaction for the patient, less expense for diagnosis and treatment, as well as future savings by delaying or preventing a disease. Their real concern is continued return: an HMO may carry a patient this year, but not the next. Thus, the HMO is reluctant to pay for the prevention of a disease process for a patient who may switch to another company at any time. These organizations are finding out that in addition to giving the patient more satisfaction now, the New Medicine physician does, in fact, practice more prevention than conventional doctors do. This will save the company more money in the long run, no matter who benefits today.

Patients and their families are becoming more knowledgeable. They have access to medical information through TV, the Internet, popular magazines, books, newsletters, and word of mouth. (Many physicians have their own websites. Mine is www.docblock.com.) Their inquiry is challenging the medical iron curtain. For instance, some patients now ask about treating hypercholesterolemia with the red yeast rice rather than conventional medications such as the statins. It may be better, safer, and less expensive than a prescription drug to lower cholesterol. This kind of change is sound and, in time, will influence the whole practice of medicine. The Chinese written character for crisis means both "danger" and "opportunity." Aptly, this medical crisis holds both the danger of a reactionary limiting of health care, as well as a revolutionary opportunity to save money and lives by working with an amalgamated system of the New Medicine. Though this is very different than the orthodox medical program most of us were taught, I feel, the New Medicine is here to stay, and in time it may find a new home outdistancing the arrows of the doubting allopathic physician.

Some established and well-seasoned aspects of healing have proven to be effective not only for decades, but centuries, and even millennia. The New Medicine physician selects what is the best from all these disciplines, using, for example, acupuncture from Chinese medicine, electromagnetic diagnosis from energy medicine, remedies from homeopathic medicine, and echinacea from herbal medicine, all in a particular patient. No system is necessarily exclusive. Some of the above may have been mentioned briefly in medical school, but usually in a derogatory sense. It is about time that we start teaching these precepts in the curriculum of all medical schools. But that is only part of the solution. Practicing physicians are resistant and practice habits are hard to change. Unfortunately, the enlightened physician is frequently ridiculed to the point that he not only loses his hospital privileges, but also at times, is economically run out of town. In the coming years the medical community and, especially, the most entrenched and pharisaical physicians will have to accept this metamorphosis. Then I and others like me, including patients and health professionals, shall live in peace and harmony as medical colleagues.

Intuitively, we understand that we are all unique. We also know we have many minute differences such as blood type, IQ, and tolerance to certain foods. In the first year or two of medical school we are taught to spend enough time in our initial encounter with a patient to get to know him or her intimately. But most physicians never spend that much time with the same patient again! With more continued one-to-one time it becomes easier to know the uniqueness of that person and to focus on how that person fits into certain diagnostic categories considering the given physical and laboratory findings. In many primary care practices lab tests are done before the patient even sees a doctor. It is not just a convenience that the initial focus is on a lab test rather than on the individual; it is a sign of the times. Why not figure out which lab tests, if any, are really needed? Then, if a lab test does not agree with a patient's diagnosis, throw out the lab test, not the patient. The point is that each person is not only psychologically, but also biologically unique!

## Normal Is Not Optimal

Lab values of personal health requirements are only rough estimates of a statistical average. Thus, they do not invariably apply to a given individual who presents with a particular symptom complex. For example, we use averages such as the RDAs for nutrition. Dr. Roger Williams spent the last forty-five years of his life studying our biochemical individuality and learning that we differ by as much as thirty-fold in our need for certain nutrients, even with the same basic weight, age, and medical history. One may need thirty times as much zinc as another, or thirty times as much B-6 or folic acid to produce a certain enzymatic reaction, based on the genetic and environmental variance of need for any given person.

Normal laboratory values are derived from testing a large number of presumably healthy individuals and plotting their laboratory results in a bell-shaped curve. Values within two standard deviations of the mean are accepted as "normal." This is a statistical term in which should, by definition, apply to 87.5 percent of the population. By my definition a value is no longer optimal when it reaches any level where risk starts to increase. This is quite different than just being in the statistical range that most doctors consider normal.

The definition of normal is also influenced by technology. Laboratory examinations have been available to patients since the ancient days of medicine. Not very sophisticated in their earliest forms, they consisted of diagnosing diabetes by tasting a patient's urine to determine the presence of sugar. Today laboratory tests range from basic bacterial cultures, to routine chemistry panels to highly complex immunologically derived processes. All are intended to determine the presence or absence of an underlying disease state. For example, in the early days of measuring cholesterol, we accepted total values as high as 300 mg/dl as normal. Once we achieved the ability to measure fractions of cholesterol, however, we began thinking of an LDL level of 160 mg/dl as normal. As we learn more about heart disease we know that we should strive to attain levels much lower than these to decrease cardiovascular risk.

Some physicians have already adjusted their interpretation of lab results to reflect optimal values. For example, an LDL level of less than 100mg/dl is considered most efficacious in decreasing cardiovascular risk. A complete cardiovascular risk panel — including homocysteine, folate, B-12, cardio-CRP, and clotting factors — provides a comprehensive picture of the patient's cardiovascular health. Even with this more detailed analysis, referring only to a range of normal results may create an illusion that the individual is fine. Many experienced physicians know that a patient on the fringes of the range is not as healthy as one in the middle. For example, a person with a potassium level of 3.5—within the normal range of 3.5 to 5—is much more likely to have a fatal heart arrhythmia than if the value was 4.2. Thus, lab results should be interpreted for optimal values that inform the individual of the possible need of dietary supplements, antioxidants, hormones and pharmaceuticals. This approach gives the knowledgeable physician more effective tools for establishing goals and managing the patient's individual health program. Do not hesitate to discuss optimal vs. normal values with your doctor.

## A Medical Decision

Most discussions of proper treatment involve the buzz phrase, *Evidence Based Medicine*. According to a book of the same name written in the 90s by Dr. Sackett, the term refers to the practice of basing medical decisions on the integration of the individual clinical experience with the best available published research. Though Sackett and his colleagues attribute this idea to a few elite French physicians in the mid 1800's, Hippocrates wrote on this very concept centuries earlier. He conducted a systemic review of each patient's condition and the current knowledge of a disease to understand and catalogue the physical signs of a dying person. He then confirmed the evidence by autopsy once the patient died.

Like most physicians, we tend to think of evidence in a strictly scientific sense. The actual definition, however— "grounds for belief"— is much broader. Thus, an acupuncturist who uses any form of previous experience that combines the individual and the knowledge of general field is practicing evidence-based medicine! Any logical conclusion is based on deductive or inductive reasoning. Either or both may be applied to a medical decision. Inductive logic, the basis of the scientific method and evidence based medicine, uses specific observations to make general conclusions. Conversely, deductive logic applies a general premise to explain specific observations. At times, a physician cannot operate exclusively within these logic paradigms. He or she must instead use anecdotal evidence or intuition to make a given medical decision. This is called clinical judgement, an innate skill instilled into a physician at birth. Great physicians are born, not made. Unfortunately, patients attended by doctors who lack this quality eventually suffer from their limitations.

**Believing is Seeing**

Physicians in the past received almost all their medical knowledge through dissecting cadavers, but this practice was halted in the second century by the Holy Roman Empire. Then, at the beginning of the Renaissance, dissections were permitted again. Prior to the prohibition anatomists, especially Galen, the most prominent of the time, said that the liver had five lobes. Thus, for the next thirteen hundred years while dissections were prohibited, his observations were authoritative. Even when dissection was reinstated and Renaissance anatomists could see for themselves, it took another thirty years to establish that the liver has, as we now know, only two lobes. In other words, believing is, sometimes, seeing what others believe to be true. This is why we should not turn our belief over to the establishment; organized and orthodox medicine is not always right! Like those early Renaissance anatomists, the establishment's indoctrination has temporarily blinded them.

Part of the New Medicine's world view is allowing the uniqueness and the complexity of the individual to teach us to rethink the role of a given statistic. Each healing system has its own diagnostic grid through which it sees a patient.

Ayurvedic, Chinese, and homeopathic medicines each look at people from a different perspective. They also have a distinct therapeutic armamentarium. Consequently, a diagnosis is relative. It is just one way of organizing facts, and each system uses a different format. With the New Medicine we have no ideological or conventional limitations; we can treat somebody with several systems of medicine at once. The primary concern is the individual. As noted earlier, the whole is greater than the sum of its parts. Understanding how those parts interact in each human being, and being willing to make use of the whole of the world's healing traditions is paramount. Wisely, it is acupuncture and drugs, not acupuncture or drugs for pain syndromes; it is light therapy and anti-depressant drugs, rather than light therapy or anti-depressant drugs to treat depression. Since the patient is a whole person, the physician takes into consideration all aspects of his or her life — physical, emotional, spiritual, familial, ethnic, economic, social, and occupational. This opens up unparalleled possibilities, both for understanding the individual and, ultimately, for helping the patient to heal him/herself. It also allows us to see beyond the limitations of what we were taught to see and truly believe in what we see for ourselves.

## Dissatisfaction Causes Disease

Many of us are tremendously dissatisfied, not only with our society, but, in particular, with our work. Part of our process of healing, whether it is from heart disease, infection, or even cancer, has to do with profoundly changing some or all aspects of our lives. For example, our workplaces, the way we work, or even the particular kind of work we do could be detrimental. As with my colleagues in their primary care medical practice, about sixty percent of my patients have serious problems with their occupations. One must deal with these issues. They are major factors in overall health. Consider an unhappy paralegal who is word-processing all day long. While she works she is cursing the boss for how much work she has to do. She is, indeed, in a stressful situation.

Much of her neuroendobiology is in overdrive, causing an internal imbalance. She will likely develop some malady such as carpal tunnel syndrome, a stiff neck, a pain in her shoulders, or lower back because she is rigid and furious. I have some patients who are writers, and none of them ever have carpal tunnel syndrome. These folks spend as much time at the word processor as the paralegal, but they like their work. Of course, not every administrative assistant gets the syndrome, but the ones I have met who do, tend to be very dissatisfied with their work. So, how can I help her? It may be vitamin B-6, acupuncture, hypnosis, or even surgery for her carpal tunnel syndrome. I am not, however, addressing the underlying problem of her dissatisfaction; I am just applying a band-aid. A good practitioner needs to consider all aspects of the patient in the whole of the healing scheme. According to a published study of men in Massachusetts in 1980, the major cause of first heart attacks was not heredity, high cholesterol, hypertension, nor smoking, but job dissatisfaction.

George Angle, a professor of medicine at the University of Rochester, wrote several books in the 1960s on the fundamental causes of illness. He looked, over a period of many years, at patients with a variety of serious illnesses such as cancer, heart disease, stroke, multiple sclerosis and Parkinson's disease. When he went back and did histories of these people he found that in the years before the onset of illness many described a sense of giving up. Eighty percent of the people who developed these serious, often life-threatening illnesses, felt they were losing, or had already lost the game of life. These patients were adults, many of them professionals, not children who could be easily influenced. When Angle went back to their families to make sure this was not some kind of retrospective bias, he confirmed his hypothesis: disease is caused by *dis-ease*. Unhappy people are prone to major illness. This conclusion is closely related to the mind-body interaction discussed earlier. We know, for example, the mind affects our immune system. A depressed immune system is fertile ground not only for infection, but also cancer. If the immune system is over-stimulated, such inflammatory diseases as rheumatoid arthritis or lupus can occur. So, in addition to conventional histories, physicals, and lab studies, a patient's condition of ease, or perspective on his or her own life needs to be considered. This is the holistic approach in the New Medicine.

Traditionally, the spiritual dimension or a spiritual advisor is mentioned only when somebody is close to dying. At that point they call in the chaplain. Otherwise, the spiritual aspect is more or less ignored and factored out of total health care. In the New Medicine, however, we do not have to abide by this taboo. I have seen faith's affect on both health and illness. In our practice we now incorporate a doctor of ministry, a healer, who joins us once or twice a week to enhance the effects of our current therapies and work with patients who do not respond to conventional treatment. My nurse and I also pray with and for our patients, and mercifully, we have seen miracles.

## Partners

This new medicine emphasizes a healing partnership. This practice is common with a psychotherapist, but not with a primary care physician. The patient and the doctor need a therapeutic alliance. The benefit of an alliance is fortification, in this context, against disease. Dr. Bernie Siegel, the famous cancer surgeon, has his patients use a combat metaphor with imaging. He asks them to see in their mind's eye the artillery of chemotherapy raining down and destroying the cancer. If they have an infection, he has them visualize the white cells amassing and invading the bacteria. In his books he gives numerous examples of how we can best image. Rather than being passive, we can learn about an illness and the vulnerable areas, and attack the disease. This mobilizes the whole human system and favorably affects the outcome. This healing partnership implies collaboration, not compliance.

In a doctor-patient relationship compliance is an ugly word. It means, "You do what I tell you to; and if you do, you are a good patient, and if you do not you are a bad patient!" I prefer to be in league with my patients. We're on the same team. As I mentioned earlier, I am the coach, he or she is the captain, and, together, the team makes the essential decisions about treatment. The patient may obtain most of the information from me, but I also urge him or her to consult other individuals, a support group, the Internet, books, and magazine articles about the illness. I encourage my patients to discuss those things with me, and I frequently learn from them. This kind of personal research is important to the partnership because a person who is completely involved with the disease, and who more or less understands the treatment, will do what is recommended with conviction, rather than out of compliance with what the doctor thinks is right. If a patient does not want to cooperate I bless him and let him go on his way, always leaving my door open. This way there is no bad blood between us. I could make the patient feel guilty, or cause him to lie to me, pretending he is doing something he is not. By coming to me freely, though, he acknowledges that something needs to be done. This is truly a partnership. As a doctor, I will do my best to help overcome the malady, but the patient has the responsibility for his disease; he owns it. At times then, a patient requests a particular therapy even when I recommend another. I am amazed sometimes that his or her choice was actually better than mine.

Unfortunately, this type of patient involvement or self-care is sadly neglected in today's medical philosophy. Self-care includes learning about ourselves, as well as taking care of ourselves so we can then expand our knowledge and help others to take care of themselves. Self-care must encompass self-awareness; we must have a sense of what is going on before we can do something about it. I ask people, "Why do you think this is happening? Why do you think you had five colds this winter when you never had more than one? Why is your blood pressure skyrocketing?" After patients get over their initial shock— "...this is what I came here to find out"— most of them can tell me that something has changed: things are terrible at home; they hate their work supervisor; they are depressed; they are eating like a pig; and so on. Whatever it might be, they do have a sense of what went wrong, and hence precipitated their medical problem.

## Thinking Can Make It So

Learning how to relax is basic to self-care. Relaxation is the antidote for stress, the fight or flight response. It is a balancing of an involuntary wrestling match of the parasympathetic versus the sympathetic nervous systems. True relaxation is a form of concentrated meditation that changes our brain waves from the *beta*, or thinking state, to the *alpha*, a rather translucent and counterpoised state. For completeness, the *theta* is the drowsy, half-asleep phase, and *delta* is the sleep state with the possibility of dreaming. If we can get ourselves into a relaxed state ten to twenty minutes twice a day, we can improve virtually every physiological function in our bodies, and, as a result, almost any clinical or mental condition. When we temporarily eliminate the mental tug of war in our daily routines and allow the body to enter a state of quiet counterpoise, our homeostasis, balance, or functional equilibrium begins to prevail. Many techniques are used to relax; several simple ones follow.

Sit comfortably in a quiet room in a chair and uncross your legs and arms to eliminate muscular tension. With feet on the floor rest the arms easily in your lap or on the arms of the chair. Close your eyes and breathe in through the nose and out through your mouth, allowing your belly to be soft. Try to keep your mind blank; listen to your minds voice "soft" as you breathe in, and "relaxed" as you breathe out. If thoughts intrude, let them come and let them go.

A mantra is the second technique that can be used. It comes from the "Transcendental Meditation" (TM) which is of sub-continental Indian origin. A mantra is a special word we select for ourselves that frequently has a harmonious vibration internally and externally. It is a word that represents harmony with the universe, like "One," "Peace" or "Love." My personal mantra is "peace." I close my eyes and every time I exhale I see peace, either the word, or the letters, p-e-a-c-e, coming out of my mouth in smoke gradually floating up, forming the word. The mantra needs to fit our personal belief systems. Thus, some choose, "Jesus," and others, "Relax." Although sleep is not part of this process, one may, after ten to fifteen minutes, fall asleep to wake up refreshed. During this period of relaxation the body rejuvenates to continue with the day. Furthermore, when a stressful situation arises, I tell my patients to utter their mantra, or for a few seconds to go through the action of their mantra, and suddenly, like Pavlov's dogs, a programmed response relaxes the individual. You might remember, Pavlov rang a bell each time he fed a group of dogs. After several days of feeding, he rang the bell and the dogs would salivate even though there was no food. This is a conditioned response that happens in most higher animals, including the highest, the human being. As the highest, we can also learn form the others; dogs know about self-care, even if their masters do not. (See "If a Dog were Your Teacher," page 52.)

A psychiatrist colleague of mine, Clancy McKenzie, M.D., whom I met at Capital University, taught me his technique of using a light level of meditation for solving problems and making decisions. In America, if big is good, bigger is better. With meditation, however, deeper levels are beneficial for some purposes, but not others.

One of the most effective states of mind is that which humans have used for a hundred thousand years. It is a slightly relaxed level of consciousness attained if one were to sit in the middle of a woods and listen, with eyes closed, to the sounds of the forest. Clearly, this is not easily acquired in urban life, with the bright lights, loud noises and pressures of modern society. Still, we have several alternatives to simulate the tranquility of a sylvan retreat.

First, sit comfortably erect, using balance rather than muscle tension. This way the spine will straighten and elongate automatically as deeper meditation is reached. Crossing one's legs at the ankles if the chair is short will distribute pressure between the feet and bottoms of the thighs.

Technically, for proper energy flow, the left ankle is behind the right. To reach an alpha state it is helpful to elevate the gaze approximately thirty degrees and close the eyes. This is not hypnosis; this is directing our mind to do what we want it to do. The next step is counting backward from ten to zero, pacing ourselves with our breathing. We inhale slowly and see, hear, or just imagine the number as we exhale. Another technique is to picture ourselves going down a flight of stairs as we count backward from ten, descending with every step. When we get to zero, or the floor at the bottom of the steps, we will be at a deeper level of consciousness. We already begin at a deeper level when we close our eyes looking up. Our total being knows how to get into this state of relaxation. Thousands of years have drawn us to the forest, to the plain, and to the hilltop. Does a fish need to learn how to swim; does a rabbit need to learn to hop, or a bird to fly? Just decide that your mind will do this, and it will.

Every time we daydream, we are close to this plane, and we pass through this and deeper levels every night when we fall asleep. Unfortunately, we do not take advantage of the opportunity to meditate then. When an amateur gets to a meditation level and starts thinking, he is no longer at that level. Meditation is a matter of getting beyond body and mind. When we move back into thought, we move out of meditation. For meditation is the now, not the past, nor the future.

This concept can be applied to give us an answer to a specific problem related to our underlying mental (subconscious) state. We formulate the question in advance and decide that the moment we reach zero, the first thing that occurs in our mind will be the answer to the question already posed. Also, we can mentally picture how we want to feel after we get our answer: happy, alert, no headache, etc. This has a powerful effect that lasts throughout the day.

The difficulty of this relaxation exercise is maintaining awareness and not falling asleep. In meditation we aim for deeper relaxation but heightened awareness. This translates into slower brain wave frequencies with greater amplitude. Thus, we must train ourselves to go two seemingly opposite directions at once. To this end I am currently researching neurofeedback, which uses an electric encephalogram hooked up to a computer that will teach us not only to enter relaxation, but also to reprogram our brains for the alpha state and deeper. With a little (assisted) practice one can do this at will. This technique has been used on thousands of youngsters with ADHD, hundreds of people with traumatic brain damage, and people like you and me who want to improve our mental lot in life.

Practicing a relaxation exercise or a mantra ten to forty-five minutes once or twice a day indeed improves one's outlook, decreases anxiety, lowers blood pressure, and enables the whole body to work better. Plainly, these procedures are useful in the absence of illness, but they can also be applied to many medical diseases. Fertility, for instance, is enhanced, heart disease decreased, and pain syndromes improved, all along with our general well being.

The words, meditation and medicine, are derived from the same Sanskrit root, meaning both "to take the measure of" and "to care for." Each of these definitions is apparent in our understanding of medicine: an illness is assessed and then treated. Meditation accomplishes these, too, only quietly and internally. It takes measure of the moment, cares only for the present. It is, by definition, the absence of neurosis, a condition of anxiety about what happened yesterday and the threat of tomorrow. In meditation, then, one experiences only the immediate; it requires being absolutely present. If thoughts come, let them go. This removes us from stress and fosters the body's own healing. Meditation is also powerful in preventing disease. As a result, it is beginning to come back into medicine.

Actually, there are three kinds of meditation. The type outlined above is concentrated meditation. Here we concentrate on breathing and/or words. Prayers like "Our Father Who Art in Heaven..." or "Hail Mary..." or "Hare Krishna, Hare Krishna..." are all examples of concentrated meditation. A second type is awareness (or mindful) meditation. This involves becoming aware of thoughts, feelings, and sensations as they arise, and consciously releasing them. A psychiatrist, for instance, might advise this for troubling emotions. The third kind is expressive meditation which is the oldest, the least used and, in some ways, the most potent. It can include dancing, shaking, twirling, drumming, and other physical expressions. Some of this occurs in religious settings, such as davening, or swaying forward and backward in Hebrew synagogue, chanting in a Catholic mass, performing the repetitive tasks of Buddhism, raising the hands toward heaven in Christian charismatic services, or speaking in tongues like the Holy Rollers. Singing, dancing, or cheering are secular examples of using one's body to express that which is internal. Even making love includes rhythmic and expressive body movements. Yoga and ti-chi are yet other examples of expressive meditation.

**Exercise is Medicine, Too**

Anaerobic or resistance exercise, such as weightlifting, is useful both therapeutically and preventatively. Aerobic exercise, which includes biking, jogging, climbing, and swimming, has been studied the most and its total health benefits are undeniable. Numerous studies have also been conducted on yoga, ti-chi, and chi-gung, which are predominantly Eastern (particularly Chinese) forms of exercise. They are shown to effectively treat and prevent every imaginable kind of illness and condition, often with mind-blowing results. One carefully randomized and controlled group of mountain climbers in Tibet was studied as they prepared for a climb. Half of the group did aerobic conditioning, and half did gentle chi-gung exercises. After three weeks those who did chi-gung were actually in better aerobic shape than those who did aerobic conditioning!

A healthy lifestyle should include exercise, whether one has asthma, arthritis, neurological or cardiac disease. The options are numerous and adaptable to virtually any condition. Exercise is particularly important to self-care. We humans were not meant to spend eight hours a day at a desk. It is not in our genetic code; we are programmed to move around. Our ancestors, both ages ago and more recently, spent most of their time in physical activities. Now the daily work tends to be repetitive and stationary. This applies to the factory, the store, the office, the classroom, and the vehicle, to name a few workplaces. Thus, we have to find ways to move around more. One of the problems for kids who are said to have attention deficit hyperactivity disorder is being made to do something utterly inhuman; for children six or seven years old sitting in class for hours a day is virtually impossible. Their natural reaction is to fidget or tune out. We can all benefit by taking a moving break and walking to the window, to the bathroom, or just around the desk.

## Medicinal Eating

Medical skeptics have said, "Let food be your medicine, and medicine your food," — in other words, put the farm in pharmacology. Though this may sound glib, they are, pragmatically, right. In addition to nutritional foods, which will be discussed in chapter three, there are many medicinal herbs we can include in our diets. Ginger for nausea, garlic for lowering blood pressure, chamomile for relaxation, and black cohosh for menopausal symptoms are just a few examples mentioned in Chapter Five. Food allergies also affect total health. Some people are acutely allergic to foods like shellfish or peanuts which cause immediately life-threatening reactions such as restricted airways or even shock. Most food allergies, however, are subtle. Using specialized laboratories such as the Great Smoky Laboratories, many New Medicine practitioners, including me, have conducted tests with very interesting results. For example, some individuals had no "allergic" problem eating wheat, but when they stopped eating it they felt better, slept more soundly, and had less respiratory illness. In the past we responded to food sensitivities with elimination diets, but now we have blood tests that target specific food irritants. Changing diets accordingly can make significant differences in diseases such as chronic fatigue syndrome, irritable bowel disease, seizure disorders, and ADHD. In migraine studies, for example, ninety-two percent of the individuals tested had noticeably fewer headaches simply by removing foods to which they were sensitive, like coffee, chocolate, lunch meats, sharp cheeses, and wine from their diets. These food intolerances can be easily identified (see page ___ for details), making medicinal eating another aspect of self-care.

### Groups

In Western biomedicine we usually think of disease as existing in an individual body. Most of the ancient healing traditions, however, understood that even though lesions or dysfunction were visible in only one person, they could be a reflection of dysfunction in the family or community. Humans are not solitary creatures; our survival as a species has always depended on at least a limited degree of cooperation; prosperity requires more. Thus, good relationships must be recreated among individuals and their communities for anyone to be healthy. Hence, we now involve the entire household, classroom, or workplace with the healing of a patient. The resulting support groups minister to those needing care as well as those giving care. Thanks to the computer (an example of our prosperity and the corresponding increase in interaction), this network has expanded to chat rooms, bulletin boards, and health clubs available on-line.

### Disease as a Teacher

We all hope to stay healthy physically, psychologically, and financially. Being gainfully employed can serve each of these desires. It's not just about making money for money's sake, or to put food on the table, or for the small and large luxuries in life, or for financial security in our old age, but about fulfilling our purpose on this earth in the river of life. Disease can interrupt the flow. But illness can also be a great teacher. It certainly gets our attention. This does not mean that we always cause our own illnesses, but it does mean that if we have a disease, we can look at it as an opportunity for transformation. For it may be a sign that we are out of balance; the particular disease may give us a clue to the imbalance. Furthermore, if we look at disease as nothing more than a misfortune, we will see ourselves as victims. If we instead look at it as an opportunity to learn and grow, then we become students of our own lives, with self-directed goals for productivity and satisfaction. In any condition of health or illness we need to validate our worth to give us a sense of fulfillment.

True fulfillment has a deeper source than financial gain; heaven itself may be reflected in our enjoyment of our work. Though it might sound lofty or idealistic, we need to perceive a calling beyond the noisy demands of daily life, something which echoes within us saying, "This is the work I am meant to do; it is my life's work." If we do not pursue this we are bound to languish mentally, spiritually, and physically. Disease may be caused by neglecting our life's purpose. For we are profoundly blessed if our avocation can be our vocation. This does not apply only to professionals or craftsmen either. Men and women who cultivate their heartfelt desires by nurturing families, relationships, careers, or any other conviction will find the same satisfaction in life. This is a process of development and of understanding who we are, what we are meant to be, and what we are doing on this planet. It is not necessarily excitement or momentary exhilaration we should seek, but contentment. This sort of indulgence improves our lives and inspires those around us. In the New Medicine we as physicians should remind our patients of this philosophy; too often the stresses of illness nearly obliterate it. So, find a physician who is sensitive to these concerns, or teach your favorite doctor to be. We can even learn from the following example; dogs seem to understand thoroughly their calling.

## If a Dog Were Your Teacher,
## You would learn...

When loved ones come home, always run to greet them.

Never pass up the opportunity to go for a joyride.

Allow the experience of fresh air and the wind in your face to be pure ecstasy.

When it's in your best interest — practice obedience.

Let others know when they've invaded your territory.

Take naps and stretch before rising.

Run, romp and play daily.

Thrive on attention and let people touch you.

Avoid biting, when a simple growl will do.

On warm days, stop to lie on your back on the grass.

On hot days, drink lots of water and lie under a shady tree.

No matter how often you're scolded, don't buy into the guilt thing and pout ... run right back and make friends.

Delight in the simple joy of a long walk.

Eat with gusto and enthusiasm.

Stop when you have had enough.

Be loyal.

Never pretend to be something you're not.

If what you want lies buried, dig until you find it.

When someone is having a bad day, be silent, sit close by and nuzzle them gently.

# THREE

# Food For Thought

## Background

Food is any organic substance used as a fuel to energize our living tissue. Our metabolism also converts it to basic building blocks that are as fundamental to our constitution as our genes. In fact, eating and drinking wisely allows us to overrule our genes. We are one of the few animals on earth that can do this. In this chapter we'll discuss the various components of food, the benefits of eating healthily, and the price we pay if we do not.

Unfortunately, gluttony has been built into our genetic code. Because of frequent famines and other conditions of scarcity, even after the development of agriculture, humans learned to overeat whenever possible. It was survival not of the fittest, but of the fattest. Now, after years of plenty, being overweight has reached epidemic proportions.

Our genes are of ancient origin — they are as much as two million years old. Research has shown that chimpanzees are only 1.6 percent different from us genetically. The collective human genome has changed only minimally since modern Homo sapiens became widespread about thirty-five thousand years ago. We are classified as omnivores, and though we eat flesh, or meat, like carnivores, our bodies are partial to being herbivores. Carnivores have claws, while herbivores have hands or hoofs. The teeth of a carnivore are sharp, but the teeth of an herbivore are mainly flat for grinding. The intestinal tract is short in a carnivore, but the human intestine is twenty-six feet long. A carnivore cools its body by panting; an herbivore sweats. The biggest difference, depending on our genetic makeup, is metabolic. Carnivores manufacture their own vitamin C. Like other herbivores we must obtain it from our diet. Furthermore, when we eat like carnivores some of us elevate certain chemicals like uric acid, lipids, and sugar in our bodies to dangerous levels, causing gout, cerebral vascular disease, and diabetes, respectively.

## Genetic Reactions to Food

Prior to the development of agriculture approximately twelve thousand years ago, we were hunters and gatherers. According to some experts, grains, dairy products, and re-fined sugars are the bane of human existence. These were not in the diet of our ancient ancestors. The meats consumed were lean, coming from wild game. Gathered foods were also low fat and high fiber. Different blood types developed in response to these food sources and lifestyles. The oldest blood type of the human race is type O. On the Savannah plains of Africa, where, according to Dr. Peter J. D'Adamo, humans developed, survival depended on intense physical exercise and animal protein. These ancient people were primarily hunters. Thus, they ate virtually no dairy products and only negligible amounts of grain. Then, through evolution and migration, blood type A developed. These humans subsisted on a vegetarian diet since they were foremost gatherers and poor hunters. Type B developed with animal husbandry and milk production. These people had strong digestive systems that could tolerate both animal and vegetable proteins. The most recent in terms of evolution is the rare type AB. Be-cause these humans are biologically more complex they can eat foods from the A group as well as the B group.

Though our lifestyle is no longer dominated by how we obtain our food, the correlation between diet and blood type is still strong. When people eat correctly for their blood type they not only feel better, but they also have fewer degenera-tive diseases (e.g., cardiovascular disease, obesity, arthritis), allergies, and cancer. It should be noted that an A, B, or O blood type has nothing to do with whether one is rh positive (e.g., O+) or negative (e.g., A-).

Our blood types are defined by their antigens. Antigens are markers, like antennae, on all of our cells that recognize foreign substances. When our specific blood type antigens detect a foreign antigen like that of a virus, bacteria, parasites, or other incompatible protein entering our system they immediately create antibodies to attack the invader. In a reaction called agglutination the antibodies glue themselves to the foreign antigen and destroy it. Nearly one hundred years ago Dr. Karl Landsteiner, a physician and scientist, discovered this reaction and revolutionized blood transfusions. We use this concept today in "Type and Cross Matching" to predetermine compatibility in the use of blood donors.

A version of this reaction also occurs with some of the foods we eat. Based on our genetically determined blood type our cells find certain lectins, or protein molecules found in foods, harmful foreign substances. These lectins have agglutinating properties and will adhere onto various cells in our bodies. For example, if one eats a food that contains a dietary protein lectin that is incompatible with his or her blood type antigen, the body reacts as if to a foreign protein. The lectins often target an organ, accumulate, and disturb cells in that tissue. If this happens in the intestines, then, perhaps, irritable bowel syndrome is experienced, if in the joints, arthritis, and so on. In other words, we can stay healthier, feel better, and conserve our energy if we do not have to fight the food we eat. The solution, then, is to avoid the lectins that agglutinate the particular cells determined by our blood type. For a list of foods to avoid accordingly, see Table 3-I (page 56). If you do not know your blood type, ask your doctor to order one the next time he or she does any blood test, or you can request it when you donate blood. Incidentally, donating blood is healthy for you and society. Most men and post-menopausal women have too much iron, which is an oxidizing mineral, in their blood. Being a donor is both altruistic and antioxidant.

The reaction described above depends on the coding of

# TABLE 3-I
# BLOOD TYPE AND FOOD TO AVOID

## TYPE O—MOST COMMON

**Meats/Seafood** — Goose, barracuda, catfish, caviar, conch, lox, octopus, pickled herring, all pork

**Eggs/Dairy** — American cheese, blue cheese, brie, buttermilk, camembert, casein, cheddar, colby, cottage cheese, cream cheese, edam, emmenthal, goat milk, gouda, gruyere, ice cream, jarlsberg, kefir, monterey jack, munster, parmesan, provolone, neufchatel, ricotta, skim or 2% milk, string cheese, swiss, whole milk, yogurt (all varieties)

**Oils/Fats/Nuts/Seeds** — Corn oil, cottonseed oil, peanut, safflower oil, brazil nuts, cashews, lichi, peanuts, peanut butter, pistachios, poppy seeds

**Beans** — Copper, kidney, navy and tamarind beans; domestic, green and red lentils

**Cereals/Bread/Grains/Pasta** — Cornflakes, cornmeal, cream of wheat, familia, farina, grape nuts, oat bran, oatmeal, seven-grain, shredded wheat, wheat bran, wheat germ, wheat bagels, corn muffins durum wheat, english muffins, high-protein bread, wheat matzos, multi-grain bread, oat bran muffins, pumpernickel, wheat bran muffins, whole wheat bread, bulgur wheat flour, coucous flour, gluten flour, graham flour, oat flour, soba noodles, semolina and spinach pasta, white and whole wheat flour

**Vegetables/Fruits** — CA avocado; brussel sprouts, chinese, red and white cabbage; cauliflower; white and yellow corn; eggplant; domestic and shitake mushrooms, mustard greens; black, greek and spanish olives; red and white potatoes; alfalfa sprouts; blackberries; coconuts; cantaloupe and honeydew melon; oranges; plantains; rhubarb; tangerines; apple juice and cider; cabbage juice; orange juice

**Spices/Condiments** — Capers; cinnamon; cornstarch; corn syrup; nutmeg; black and white pepper; apple cider, balsamic, red wine and white vinegar; ketchup; dill, kosher, sweet and sour pickles; relish

**Beverages** — Coffee, distilled liquor, sodas, black tea.

## TYPE A — COMMON

**Meats/Fish/Seafood** — Beef, buffalo, duck, goose, heart, lamb, liver, mutton, partridge, pheasant, all pork, rabbit, veal, venison, quail, anchovy, barracuda, beluga, bluefish, bluegill, bass, catfish, caviar, clam, conch, crab, crayfish, eel, flounder, frog, gray sole, haddock, haka, halibut, herring (fresh or pickled), lobster, lox, mussels, octopus, oysters, scallop, shad, shrimp, sole, squid, striped bass, tilefish, turtle

**Eggs/Dairy** — American cheese, blue cheese, brie, butter, buttermilk, camembert, casein, cheddar, colby, cottage, cream cheese, edam, emmenthal, gouda, gruyere, ice cream, jarlsberg, monterey jack, munster, neufchatel, parmesan, provolone, sherbet, skim or 2% milk, sour cream (non-fat), swiss, whole milk

**Oils/Fats/Nuts/Seeds** — Corn, cottonseed oil, peanut, safflower oil; brazil nuts, cashews, pistachios

**Beans** — Copper, garbanzo, kidney, lima, navy, red, tamarind

**Cereals/Bread/Grains/Pasta** — Cream of wheat, familia, farina, granola, grape nuts, wheat germs, seven grain, shredded wheat, wheat bran, durum wheat, english muffins, high-protein bread, wheat matzos, pumpernickel, wheat bran muffins, whole wheat bread, whole wheat and white flour, semolina pasta, spinach pasta

**Vegetables/Fruits** — Chinese, red and white cabbage; eggplant; domestic and shitake mushrooms; black, greek and spanish olives; green, red, yellow and jalapeno peppers; sweet, red and white potatoes; yams; tomatoes; bananas; coconuts; mangoes; cantaloupe and honeydew melon; oranges; papayas; plantains; rhubarb; tangerines; orange juice; papaya juice; tomato juice

**Spices/Condiments** — Capers; gelatin; black, cayenne, peppercorn, red and white pepper; apple cider, balsamic, red or white vinegar; wintergreen; ketchup; mayonnaise; tabasco, worcestershire sauce

**Beverages** — Beer, liquor, sodas, black tea (regular or decaffeinated)

## TYPE B — RARE

**Meats/Fish/Seafood** — Chicken, cornish hens, duck, goose, heart, partridge, all pork, quail, anchovy, barracuda, beluga, bluegill, bass, clam, conch, crab, crayfish, eel, farm-raised salmon, frog, lobster, lox, mussels, octopus, oysters, sea bass, shrimp, snail, striped bass, turtle, yellowtail

**Eggs/Dairy** — American cheese, blue cheese, ice cream, string cheese

**Oils/Fats/Nuts/Seeds** — Canola oil, corn oil, cottonseed oil, peanut oil, safflower oil, sesame oil, sunflower oil, cashews, filberts, pignola, pistachio, peanuts, peanut butter, poppy seeds, pumpkin seeds, sesame butter and seeds, tahini, sunflower seeds

**Beans** — Aduke; azuki; black; garbanzo; pinto; domestic, green and red lentils; black-eyed peas

**Cereals/Bread/Grains/Pasta** — Amaranth, barley, buckwheat, cornflakes, cornmeal, cream of wheat, kamut, kasha, rye, seven-grain, shredded wheat, wheat bran, wheat germ, wheat bagels, corn muffins, durum wheat, multi-grain bread, 100% rye bread, rye crisp, rye vita, wheat bran muffins, whole wheat floor, buckwheat, coucous, gluten flour, soba noodles

**Vegetables/Fruits** — Domestic and jerusalem artichoke, CA avocado, white and yellow corn; black, green, greek and spanish olives; pumpkin, radishes, sprouts, tempeh, tofu, tomato, coconuts, persimmons, pomegranate, prickly pear, rhubarb, starfruit, mung sprouts

**Spices/Condiments** — Allspice, almond extract, barley malt, cinnamon, cornstarch, corn syrup, ketchup, plain gelatin, black ground and white pepper, tapioca, all spices; capers

**Beverages** — Distilled liquor, sodas

## TYPE AB — — — VERY RARE

**Meats/Fish/Seafood** — Beef, buffalo, chicken, cornish hens, duck, goose, heart, partridge, all pork, venison, quail, anchovy, barracuda, beluga, bluegill, bass, clam, conch, crab, crayfish, eel, farm-raised salmon, flounder, frog, gray sole, haddock, halibut, pickled herring, lobster, lox, octopus, oysters, sea bass, shrimp, striped bass, turtle, yellowtail

**Eggs/Dairy** — American cheese, blue cheese, brie, butter, buttermilk, camembert, ice cream, parmesan, provolone, sherbet, whole milk

**Oils/Fats/Nuts/Seeds** — Corn oil, cotton seed oil, peanut oil, safflower oil, sesame oil, sunflower oil, filberts, poppy seeds, pumpkin seeds, sesame seeds, tahini, sunflower seeds

**Beans** — Aduke; azuki; black; fava, garbanzo; kidney; lima; black-eyed peas

**Cereals/Bread/Grains/Pasta** — Buckwheat, corn, kamut, kasha, corn muffins, artichoke pasta, soba noodles

**Vegetables/Fruits** — Domestic and jerusalem artichoke, CA avocado, white and yellow corn; abalone and shitake mushrooms, black olives, green and red and yellow peppers, jalapeno peppers, radishes, radish sprouts, mung sprouts, bananas, coconuts, guava, mangoes, oranges, persimmons, pomegranate, prickly pear, rhubarb, starfruit

**Spices/Condiments** — Allspice, almond extract, anise, barley malt, capers, cornstarch, corn syrup; black, cayenne pepper (black, cayenne, red flakes, peppercorn), tapioca, vinegar (balsamic, red or white), ketchup, pickles (kosher, sweet, sour), relish, worcestershire sauce

**Beverages** — Distilled liquor, sodas, black tea

*(If appropriate, xerox and cut out your blood type to carry in your wallet.)*

56

our red blood cell type. As mentioned earlier, this is not technically an allergic reaction. A true food allergy originates in the white blood cells (lymphocytes) and internal lining cells. If one eats a food against which the body has developed a specific antibody group, an explosive reaction takes place. This results in acute inflammation of the skin, nerves, or more serious, sudden reduction of the airways, or anaphylactic shock (cardiovascular pulmonary collapse), which is occasionally lethal. Shellfish, certain nuts, and strawberries are the most common offenders of this sort, and must be completely avoided by people allergic to them.

Food intolerances are also the result of bodily incompatibility, but they usually do not call as much attention to themselves. Lactose, sugar, and wheat/gluten intolerances are now well accepted medical diagnoses. Other hidden food intolerances are not as well accepted, but are nevertheless important in a holistic physician's thinking. They do not cause discernible immediate reactions, but over time subtle symptoms gradually build up. Obesity and degenerative diseases are attributed to this phenomenon, as are acne, stuffy nose, irritable bowel, recurrent respiratory infection, migraines, achy muscles, ADHD, and fatigue.

Methodically eliminating individual foods is the do-it-yourself method of identifying specific food intolerances. This, however, is time-consuming and can be frustrating to someone who has identified the problem but not its source. Fortunately there is an easier way: blood tests can detect the offending food. The best of these, the ALCAT (Antigen Leukocyte Cellular Antibody Test) is now offered by several laboratories, including the Great Smokies Laboratories (phone 800-522-4762), and American Medical Testing Laboratories (phone 800-881-AMTL). Information is also available on the web at www.alcat.com. After eliminating the culprit(s) from your diet you will see amazing improvements in your health. Phenolics, a configuration of a ring of hydrocarbons, is found in as many as one third of our amino acids. These do cause a subtle allergy in many people who consume them as food coloring or flavor, causing a host of symptoms from a nonspecific rash to epilepsy. Rather than discovering and eliminating the offending agent, a dilute preparation of several of these chemicals is made. Taking under the tongue on an empty stomach, thirty percent of these folks are markedly improved after three weeks. The Dessert Corp in Utah is one such organization that makes this preparation. Again beware; most orthodox physicians call this rubbish, but stand your ground and find a sympathetic doctor.

## The Skinny on Fat

Apart from glamorized cultural, advertising, and stellar body images we have medical standards of appropriate weight. Thus, when patients ask me, "What should I weigh?" we discuss their Ideal Weight, the Body Mass Index (BMI) which relates size to weight in a numerical value, percent body fat, and Waist to Hip Ratio (WHR). The ideal BMI is less than 25; the ideal percent body fat is fifteen percent for males and twenty-two percent for females; and the WHR is less than 1.0 for a man, and .85 for a woman. Though these may sound like aesthetic measurements, they are not. Excessive abdominal girth, for instance, is associated with metabolic abnormalities that cause both morbidity (illness) and mortality (death). Alternatively, we can assess our weight ourselves by standing naked in front of a long mirror. A female at her ideal weight will have little cellulite and no fat rolls, and a male should see his ribs without having love handles below them.

According to recent literature, thirty-three percent of adults do not pass this test. In some populations such as Hispanics or the Pima Indians, as many as sixty percent are overweight. Certainly, the agricultural and industrial revolutions have given society more food and less physical work than we need. Eating too much is only part of the problem. Being overweight or, in some cases, obese has both genetic and environmental causes. Paradoxically, when one is over the age of seventy, having excess weight may not be so bad. In an article in the *Archives of Internal Medicine* (Vol. 160: Sep 25, 2000; 2641-2644), patients hospitalized with a

BMI of greater than 25 had a better outcome than those less than 25.

The mindset of our society and, unfortunately, of many physicians is, "If fat does not pass my lips, it will not end up on my hips." While it is true that fat is a highly caloric food, it is actually carbohydrates that make us fat! Research shows that the prevalence for being overweight rose from 25.4 percent in 1976 to 33.3 percent in 1988—a thirty-one percent increase! During the same period the average fat intake adjusted for total calories dropped five percent. Therefore, reduced fat intake and the frequent consumption of low calorie food products is paradoxically associated with an increase of obesity. Best-sellers such as *Sugar Busters, Protein Power, Dr. Atkin's New Diet Revolution, Neanderthin,* and *The Zone* have tried to remedy this by recommending low-carbohydrate diets. This does not imply that eating fat indiscriminately is harmless. Fat has nine calories per gram while protein and carbohydrates have only four. Still, scientists believe that ninety percent of our excess carbohydrates go directly into unsightly storage rather than being burned for fuel.

Furthermore, we do not burn enough calories with regular exercise. Because of modern transportation, communications, and other labor saving inventions of the last three centuries, our daily lives require less muscle use than in the past. Thus, to stay healthy some of us do artificial work, deliberate exercise, to make up for our lack of useful physical activity. Aerobic exercise, the sustained use of muscles for twenty to thirty minutes, is good. But anaerobic or resistance exercise like lifting weights and working with a Nautilus-like machine is better.

According to a study presented at The Experimental Biology meeting in New Orleans on April 7, 1997, a virus (adenovirus AD-36) might also increase the risk of obesity and may even be contagious! Reportedly, fifteen percent of overweight people at the University of Wisconsin Obesity Clinic had antibodies to this virus, while none of the lean individuals did. Despite the possibility that obesity could be virally induced, genetically programmed, or developed by work saving machines, we do not have to be overweight or obese. Proper eating practices alone can override these influences, because how much we eat is often determined by how we eat. We need to practice tasting and appreciating our food. If we relax briefly before sitting down and eat without distractions such as television, we might enjoy the food more. It is also recommended to start a meal with a glass of water or a bowl of soup to fill the stomach and allow us to eat less. Anticipating something pleasant after the meal lures us away from the table and lingering to eat as long as the food exists. Eating controlled portions of food served on small individual plates discourages helping ourselves from a large platter "family style." In our land of plenty the adage, "waste not, want not" does not apply. We should feel no guilt when leaving food on our plate to be thrown away: it is less wasteful to throw food in the garbage than it is to eat it when we do not need to.

The sensation of hunger is linked to a recently discovered hormonal pathway. The hypothalamus (in the brain) produces a hormone called neuropeptide-Y3. This hormone drives us to eat and, at the same time, slows our metabolism. This slowing increases insulin, causing us to burn fewer calories. This in turn stimulates our adrenal gland to make cortisone, which raises the blood sugar and causes weight and fluid gain. Glucose (sugar) is then stuffed into our fat cells as fat rather than being burned by our muscles.

Another key hormone is leptin, not to be confused with lectin, the protein antigen of food. When this is released by our fat cells it tells our brain we have had enough to eat. Unfortunately, the lower the calorie intake, or the more calories burned by exercise, the less leptin is produced, making it harder to lose weight. This is part of the body's response to aging. It affects women earlier, but as we get older the sexes have the same propensity to hold on to their extra pounds. Thus, to most of us, losing weight seems like a losing battle. To make matters worse, the mind becomes preoccupied with food due to these supra-hormonal changes. Leptin injections may be a possibility, although research shows they cause fertility decrease. Certain hormones, such as thyroid, cortisone, and serotonin play a role in obesity. We also know that other hormones, like the adrenal sub-hormone called Beta-3, stimulate specific fat cells referred to as "brown fat" and powerfully affect weight-control.

In the 1890s sanitized tapeworms were used for promoting weight loss (see page 24), but now we use prescription medications or over-the-counter remedies and preparations. Phenteramine is the mainstay of treatment. It is inexpensive (fifteen cents a day), and taken only once daily, but has a slight liability for addiction. The several generics on the market may be as good as the brand name, Ionamin™, and much cheaper. I recommend the blue one with the micro globules rather than the yellow one. I have had some success with Meridia, which is much more expensive (three dollars a day), but less addictive than Phenteramine. It works like Phen/Fen, which was taken off the market for causing heart valve abnormalities. Another drug with a different mechanism is Orlastat (Xenical®). It deactivates the enzyme lipase in the intestine. The fat goes in one end and comes out the other since it is not absorbed. One can lose five hundred calories a day with this drug alone, taken before each meal in a 120 mg dose. In a way, this drug is a deterrent from eating rich food (which is usually high in fat). For if we do, there will be grumbling in the abdomen, diarrhea, and in some cases, soiling of underclothes. At times physicians combine several drugs in the same patient and, as such, might prescribe Phen/Xen (Phenteramine/Xenical). Some of the diabetic drugs do help with the weight loss and are starting to be used. In particular, those that promote insulin sensitivity are Actos™ and Avandia™, and better yet, Glucophage™. The latter drug also causes some loss of appetite, as well as promoting less glucose release by the liver. Cimetadine (Tagamet) is available without a prescription, or less expensive with a prescription. This drug is given in a 400 mg dose to be taken one hour before a meal. Cimetadine also helps in nocturnal binge eating. Some poor folks consume more than half of their calories after their evening meal. Twelve designer drugs are waiting to come out, including leptin. These drugs do everything from changing the involved obesity hormone to giving us exercise in a pill.

Obesity is a more complex condition than being overweight; it is, in fact, a disease. It is not merely lack of will power, slovenliness, or gluttony, but a neuro- hormonal imbalance, genetically endowed and environmentally nurtured. Obesity is actually the most common form of malnutrition in our modern society, resulting from an improper complement of macro- and micronutrients. According to the law of natural thermodynamics, if we ingest more calories than we can burn off, we store the excess in the form of fat. Excess fat is mentally and physically destructive. Obese people have a much higher incidence of degenerative diseases such as cardiovascular and metabolic disease (diabetes, gout, etc.), arthritis, and cancer, especially of the colon, breast, and uterus.

In morbidly obese refractory cases in which the individual has yo-yoed many times I do recommend surgery. Bypass procedures such as hooking the stomach to the lower part of the small intestine by sewing a small pouch of the stomach, and short-cutting most of the upper part of the small intestines are the usual procedures. Gastric banding has been done with laparotomy for the last forty years, a major surgery through an incision in the abdomen. This is now possible with laproscopy, a less invasive procedure used in Europe for the last three years, virtually on an outpatient basis. An inflatable pouch is inserted through a small keyhole in the abdomen. Its volume can then be adjusted as needed with a needle placed through the skin to enlarge or decrease the stomach volume.

For now, there is no magic to weight loss, but everyone can lose by following the right guidelines: go easy on carbohydrates, eat slowly, only until you are satisfied rather than stuffed, and do not skip meals. Six small meals are better than one large meal for weight control. Most importantly, we must exercise. Resistance exercises such as weight lifting are better than aerobic exercises like walking, running, or biking. The Law of Natural Thermodynamics is simple and clear: if we burn more calories than we consume, we will lose weight.

## Flax Facts

Flaxseeds have long been valued for their health benefits (Hippocrates used flax as a remedy for gastrointestinal problems), but only recently have researchers investigated their helpful compounds. Flax is one of the best plant-based sources of alpha-linolenic acid, which the body converts to the same heart-protective omega-3 fatty acids found in salmon, sardines, and mackerel. It also contains both soluble and insoluble fiber (about three grams of total fiber per tablespoon), which promote intestinal health. In addition, flaxseed is one of the richest dietary sources of lignans, thought to protect against cancer of the breast, prostate, and colon.

I recommend one or two tablespoons of ground flaxseed a day to anyone who wants to be and stay healthy. Women experiencing menopausal or pre-menopausal symptoms should also give flax a try to help ease hot flashes and heavy bleeding, and because it may promote health of vaginal tissues. Flax is safe for almost everyone, but its mild laxative effect may bother people with inflammatory bowel disease.

Whole flax seeds are sold inexpensively at natural-food stores. Grind a quarter-cup or so at a time, in a blender or an inexpensive electric coffee grinder dedicated to flax. You must grind the tiny, hard-shelled seeds or they will pass through the body undigested. Ground flax meal should be refrigerated in an airtight opaque container, where it will keep for up to thirty days. You will know that flax meal has spoiled if it smells like paint; the flax oil has changed to linseed oil.

Flax meal has a sweet nutty flavor and tastes delicious sprinkled over cereals, soups, salads, and rice. One can also bake flax meal into muffins or bread — but bear in mind that when flax is heated it is more susceptible to spoilage. Prepared foods made from flax are becoming more common, but it can be hard to tell from the ingredients label if these products contain flax meal rather than whole seeds (which offer fewer benefits).

I don't recommend using flaxseed oil available in liquid form or in capsules. Aside from being more expensive and less palatable than flax meal, flax oil spoils faster and, most importantly, lacks the protective lignans found in the ground seeds. Peanut oil has also come into its own as a preventative to cardiovascular disease; it is as effective as olive oil. Commercially made peanut butter, however, may be hydrogenated and contain the bad trans-saturated fatty acids. Making natural peanut butter from our own peanuts is far healthier. Avocados, which are seed foods, also have wonderfully healthy oil, as do macadamia nuts and pecans. Even tiny mustard seeds have recently been touted to lower triglycerides and elevate the good HDL cholesterol.

Irish steel-cut oats are extremely popular right now. Rolled oats, which have been softened by steam and flattened by rollers to form flakes, are the most common type of oatmeal. In contrast, steel-cut oats are small round nuggets. They do take longer to cook, but because of their hardy, chewy texture they are much in demand and therefore more expensive. Still, there is essentially no difference in the fiber and nutrient content of rolled and steel-cut oats. It is, however, far better to use old-fashioned oats that have the husk on them (and more fiber) than "quick" or "instant" oats. Uncle Sam's cereal contains unprocessed oats as well as flax seeds, but these are whole.

## Macronutrients

There are only three macronutrients which will be discussed in great detail later in the chapter: I – Fats, II – Protein, III – Carbohydrates. If taken in the proper proportions, we can obtain our ideal shape and weight for our genes (or jeans, if you prefer). Although, the proportion of each has been argued vigorously by nutritionists, physicians, and scientists for hundreds of years. According to The American Heart Association, fat was supposed to be the villain, and to some of my colleagues it still is. I, like many other experts, such as Ray Audette, who in 1999 published *Neanderthin*, think it is not fat, but carbohydrates that primarily cause weight gain and subsequent poor health. Dr. Barry Sears stated that the proper proportions of a healthy diet are 40-30-30 (carbohydrates, protein, fats). Dr. Atkin asserts that we should allow only twenty percent. Dr. Michael Eads thinks sixty percent of our food should be protein. All these viewpoints can certainly cause confusion. I prefer the middle ground of Dr. Sears, who published his first of three books, *The Zone*, in 1996. Go back to basics and eat and work like a caveman to achieve a lean, strong healthy body and soul. To this I would add that the sources of the macronutrients should correspond to our blood type and accommodate our food intolerances. This personalized amalgamation of diets helps us feel better, discourages weight gain, decreases allergies, and gives us more energy. The less prepared the food and the less cooked, the better. Raw vegetables do contain enzymes easily destroyed in cooking.

**Food Labels**

Since consumers get most of their nutrition information from food labels, the Food and Drug Administration (FDA), in 1998, revised the food labeling. Before the new regulations were enacted, approximately sixty percent of processed foods had labels, but few fresh foods did. Now nutrition labeling appears on virtually all packaged foods. Only a few items, such as spices and restaurant food need not provide nutrition labels. Thanks to consumer advocacy groups and the NLEA (Nutritional Labeling Educational Act) started during this past decade, the list of ingredients for menu items is available from some restaurant management. The FDA has also established voluntary guidelines for non-packaged items such as commonly consumed fruits, vegetables, and seafood. Nutrition information for these items may be presented either in brochures or on signs posted at the point of purchase. Organic on a label means that the food was not genetically modified, irradiated to kill bacteria, fertilized by sewage sludge, not treated with hormones, antibiotics, or certain pesticides. Farmers have to mid-2002 to comply.

# Figure 3-I

# Example of a Food Label

The serving size and number of servings per container must be listed.

The package must display the product name.

The nutrition information panel provides quantities of nutrients per serving in both actual amounts and as "% of Daily Values" based on a 2000 calorie energy intake.

The ingredients must name the ingredients in descending order of predominance by weight.*

The package may make a certain approved health claims if the claims are backed by scientific researched.

The package may use decriptive terms if the product meets specific criteria.

The name and address of the manufacturer must appear on all packages

The package must always tell you the weight or measure.

*Significiance to you, the consumer what appears first is present in the largest quantity.

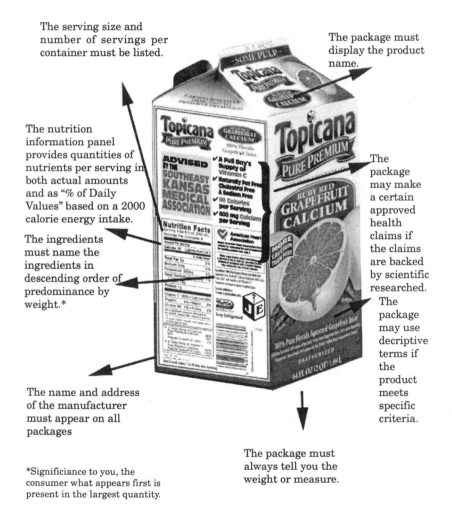

See pages 92, 93, and 294 for author's opinion on this product.

## Table 3-II
## Interpretation of Industry Jargon

**Fresh:** not previously frozen, not processed, and contains no preservatives nor additives.

**Low fat:** generally, the product contains no more than 3 grams of fat per serving (for meat, not more than 10 percent fat by weight; for milk, no more than 2 percent fat by weight).

**Low calorie:** contains fewer than 40 calories per serving or at least 1/2 the calories of the original version.

**Low cholesterol:** contains less than 20 milligrams per serving or 75 percent less cholesterol than original version.

**Natural:** contains no additives.

**Light or lite:** contains at least 25 percent less fat, sodium, or calories than original product.

**Fat free:** contains less than .5 grams of fat per serving.

**Low sodium:** contains no more than 140 milligrams of sodium per serving.

**Salt free:** contains no more than 5 milligrams of salt per serving.

## Government Rules

According to law, every prepared food label must prominently display and express in ordinary words
- The common name of the product;
- The name and address of the manufacturer, packer, or distributor;
- The net contents in terms of weight, measure, or count;
- The ingredient list;
- The serving size and number of quantities per containment;
- The quantities of specified nutrients and food constituents.

## Food Labels

◆ *Nutrition information:* a list of amounts of specific nutrients in foods.
◆ *Health message:* statements on reducing the risk, or forestalling the premature onset of certain chronic diseases through changes in diet, and only when established scientifically, such as the effects of:
- Calcium on osteoporosis
- Saturated fat and cholesterol on coronary heart disease
- Dietary fat on cancer
- Fiber contained in grain products, fruits, and vegetables on cancer and coronary heart disease
- Fruits and vegetables on cancer

### The R Trio
✔ *U.S. RDA:* United States Recommended Daily Allowances. The U.S. RDA were used on labels from the late 1960s to the early 1990s; in general, they are based on the 1968 RDA and reflect the highest RDA for any age and sex group for each nutrient.
✔ *Daily Values:* reference values developed by the FDA specifically for food labels. The Daily Values represent two sets of standards: Reference Daily Intakes (RDI) and Daily Reference Values (DRV).
✔ *Reference Daily Intake (RDI):* food labeling values for protein, vitamins, and minerals based on the RDA.
✔ *Daily Reference Values (DRV):* food labeling values for nutrients and food components (such as fat and fiber) that do not have an RDA value, but do have an important relationship with health.

## Terms on Food Labels

### GENERAL TERMS
**Free:** nutritionally trivial and unlikely to have a physiological consequence; synonyms include "without," "no," and "zero."
**High:** twenty percent or more of the Daily Value for a given

nutrient per serving.

**Less:** at least twenty-five percent less of a given nutrient than the comparison food (see individual nutrients below); synonyms include "fewer" and "reduced."

**Light or Lite:** any use of the term other than as defined below must specify what it is referring to, for example, "light in color" or "light in texture."

**Low:** an amount that would allow frequent consumption of a food without exceeding the dietary guidelines (see individual nutrients below). A food that is naturally low in a nutrient may make such a claim, but only as it applies to all similar foods. For example: fresh cauliflower, a low-sodium food"; synonyms include "little," "few" and "low source of."

**More:** at least ten percent more of a given nutrient than the comparison food; synonyms include "added."

**Good source of:** product provides between ten and nineteen percent of the Daily Value for a given nutrient per serving.

## CHOLESTEROL

**Note:** foods containing more than 13 g total fat per serving or per 50 g must indicate those contents immediately after a cholesterol claim. As we will see, all cholesterol claims are prohibited when the food contains more than 2 g saturated fat per serving.

**Cholesterol-free:** less than 2 mg cholesterol per serving and 2 g or less saturated fat per serving.

**Low in cholesterol:** 20 mg or less per serving and 2 g or less of saturated fat per serving.

**Less cholesterol:** twenty-five percent or less cholesterol than the comparison food (reflecting a reduction of at least 20 mg per serving), and 2 g or less saturated fat per serving.

## ENERGY

**Calorie-free:** fewer than five calories per serving.

**Light:** one third fewer calories than the comparison food.

**Low calorie:** less than forty calories per serving.

# FAT

**Extra lean:** less than 5 g of fat, 2 g of saturated fat, and 95 mg of cholesterol per serving and per 100 g of food.

**Fat free:** less than 0.5 g of fat per serving (and no added fat or oil).

**Lean:** Less than 10 g of fat, 4 g of saturated fat, and 95 mg of cholesterol per serving and per 100 g of food.

**Less fat:** twenty-five percent or less fat than the comparison food.

**Less saturated fat:** twenty-five percent or less saturated fat than the comparison food.

**Low fat:** 3 g or less fat per serving.

**Low saturated fat:** 1 g or less saturated fat per serving.

**Percent fat-free:** may be used only if the product meets the definitions of low fat or fat-free and must reflect the amount of fat in 100 g.

**Light:** fifty percent or less of the fat than the comparison food. For example: 50 percent less fat than regular cookies.

# FIBER

**High fiber:** twenty percent or more of the Daily Value for fiber; a high-fiber claim made on a food that contains more than 3 g fat per serving and per 100 g of food must also declare total fat.

# SODIUM

**Sodium-free and salt-free:** less than 5 mg of sodium per serving.

**Low sodium:** less than 140 mg per serving.

**Light:** a low-calorie, low-fat food with a fifty percent reduction in sodium.

**Light in sodium:** no more than fifty percent of the sodium of the comparison food.

**Very low sodium:** less than 35 mg per serving.

# SUGAR

**Sugar-free:** less than 0.5 g per serving.

Please understand that a huge discrepancy remains between oversized restaurant portions of food and the USDA recommended portions, which, in calorie portions, have increased significantly in the past decade. It seems that every restaurant tries to outdo its competitor by "giving more for the money." The article "All You Can Eat" in the March 1998 issue of *Quillon* points out that this is actually doing us a disservice rather than a service.

## I. FATS

The right fats in the right amounts are good for us. According to a Harvard health study recently published in *The Journal of The American Medical Association*, there was an inverse association between dietary fats and development of stroke in men. Why do we need fat? First, it causes the secretion of CCK (cholecyctokin) that stops the hunger sensation. We also need fat as an essential element in our metabolism. Our bodies cannot make certain fats which are referred to as *essential fatty acids*. Eicosanoids, or prostaglandins (our major chemical transmitter), HDL, cholesterol, hormones, brain tissue, and membranes lining every cell of the body are composed of fat molecules. Furthermore, we need fat for some insulation, energy stores, and most importantly, for life itself—a drastic decrease of what is known as "brown fat" is directly correlated with death. Fats also make food more palatable. However, all fats are not created equal. They range from the excellent, the good, the bad, to the very bad.

### The Good, the Bad and the Ugly

**Excellent:**
1. **Omega 3's** (DHA, EPA) in fish oils and flax.
2. **Gamalinolenic Acid** (GLA) in oatmeal, mother's milk, evening primrose oil, and borage oil. (Omega 3's + GLA increase the good ecosinoids).
3. **Alpha Linoleic Acid (ALA)** in flax and soybeans
4. **B Sitostanol.** Plant source — lowers cholesterol and possibly reduces prostate size and risk of cancer.

**Good:**
1. **Monounsaturated fats.** These are actually neutral, but not nearly as beneficial as the above. The richest source is in macadamia nuts, but it's also found in other nuts such as pistachios, walnuts, cashews and almonds as well as avocados. Olives and their oil, canola oil, and to a lesser extent, peanuts and their oil have monounsaturated fats also.
2. **Non-absorbable fats** such as Simplese® and Olestra® do not help the system, but do not hurt it either.
3. **Egg Yolks.** The yolk does contain cholesterol, but recent literature indicates it is not the cholesterol we eat, but the cholesterol our body produces in response to what we eat is bad.

**Bad:**
1. **Polyunsaturates** such as corn oil or safflower seed oil are referred to by nutritionists as Omega 6 fatty acids. They have much cis fatty acids.
2. **Saturated fats**, found in meats.

**Very Bad:**
1. Overheated oils (free radicals)
2. Hydrogenated vegetable oil, those containing the trans polyunsaturates that directly promote atherosclerosis.
3. Homogenized milk.

## THE FATS OF LIFE

The trans/cis fatty acid data is now well established. A landmark study published in *The New England Journal of Medicine* demonstrated that the consumption of products low in *trans-fatty* acids, the opposite of *cis-fatty* acids, will reduce cholesterol and triglycerides. Trans-fatty acids are partially and fully hydrogenated fats, literally from another world. They are man-made with catalysts such as nickel in the presence of hydrogen and our bodies do not know how to metabolize them. Though they are truly a *trans*-gression, they have been approved by the FDA as "a safe food additive."

Also bad are liquid oils heated to excess. This decomposes the oils and makes them into free radical-like particles. They are directly absorbed by the intestines and immediately enter the blood stream, affecting the lining of blood vessels, causing a build-up of cholesterol plaque.

On the other hand, numerous studies have shown that consuming fish which contain Omega 3's decreases the incidents of heart attacks and strokes. The Eskimo Paradox studied almost fifty years ago is a revealing testimony of this. Though their diet was overly rich in fatty foods, including animal fat (blubber and seal meat) and fatty fish, such as salmon, the Eskimos had healthy cardiovascular systems. The enigma resolved when we began to understand the strong impact of marine oils on health.

Marine oils are among the seventeen essential fatty acids which must be consumed since our bodies can make only minimal amounts (see Table 3-III). Fish oils protect the lining of the blood vessels from building up plaque, reduce triglycerides, decrease clotting, and improve the rheology (flow) of blood. They also play important roles outside the cardiovascular system in brain functioning, neurotransmitters, the retina, and improving the interaction of almost every cell in our bodies. A double-blind study published in *The Archives of General Psychiatry* in 1999 (56:407-412) showed ninety-six grams of fish oil greatly improved Bipolar (manic-depressive) Disorder. The cellular membrane (the substance that keeps the inside of the cell inside and functioning) is composed mostly of these essential fatty acids. Also, the lining of our joints and our skin are kept healthy by these Omega 3's.

As a supplement, one needs two capsules of the Omega 3's a day. Each capsule usually contains 500 mg of DHA (docosahexaenoic acid) and 200 mg of EPA (eicosapentaenoic acid) with a little Vitamin E to keep the oils fresh and provide the additional Vitamin E that is needed when these oils are consumed. One can also obtain these healthy Omega

3's the old-fashioned way by eating fish. In one study this not only preserved general health, but also prevented death from cardiovascular disease (C.M. Albert, et al. "Fish Consumption and The Risk of Sudden Cardiac Death." *JAMA* 1998; 279:23-28). Some fish contain more of these healthy fats than others. The deep cold water ocean fish with the darker flesh have the most of these life-saving oils. (See Table 3-IV.) Mackerel, salmon, and herring, for instance, are far better than catfish, orange roughy, or sole. Shellfish, such as oysters and clams, were once thought to be bad for humans because they are high in cholesterol, but are now considered safe in our metabolism since they contain many Omega 3's and another benign cholesterol-like product. Be aware, though, that these shellfish may contain a more serious health threat: various viruses which not only cause simple stomach upsets, but sometimes even death. Crustacean shellfish such as shrimp and lobster are much safer and just as healthy.

## TABLE 3-III
## DIETARY SOURCE OF OMEGA 3's

| Food Source | Omega-3 Fatty Acids per 100 g Serving |
| --- | --- |
| Atlantic mackerel | 2.5 g |
| Salmon | 1.2-1.4 g |
| Canned sardine | 1.7 g |
| Eel | 1.7 g |
| Herring | 1.6 g |
| Bluefish | 1.2 g |
| Squid | 0.9 g |
| Striped bass | 0.8 g |
| Rainbow trout | 0.5-1.0 g |
| Tuna | 0.3 g |
| Flounder | 0.2 g |

Cholesterol consumption is not that bad. In reality, it is the cholesterol that our body produces rather than what we eat that is bad for our blood vessels. Some foods villainized for their cholesterol content also have important health properties. In addition to egg yolks, cholesterol is found in all animal muscle, fowl, fish, red meats and most dairy products.

There is, for example, a sunny side to eggs. Though the egg has been maligned in the last two decades, a recent issue of *The Journal of the American Medical Association* states that an egg a day is unlikely to cause any cardiovascular problems. It raises our good as well as bad cholesterol only minimally. More importantly, it has the highest content of cystine, an important sulfur-containing amino acid. Riboflavin and niacin are found in the egg white, as is a natural source of vitamin A and E. Until 1995 it was thought that the egg had 300 mg of cholesterol in the yolk. That was the total day's allowable intake of cholesterol according to the American Heart Association. Certainly, if our diet contained this much cholesterol coming from meat, it would also contain saturated fatty acids which could elevate the bad cholesterol. We now know that an egg has 200 to 220 mg of cholesterol. In the last several years organic and nutritionally enhanced eggs have become available. A natural compound, which used to come from earthworms that our grandmothers' chickens ate, now comes from a marine algae that is fed to the chickens to produce the healthy eggs with the rich orange yolk. The organic eggs are produced by chickens who, unlike the "egg factory" chickens, are never given hormones, artificial color, antibiotics, or pesticides. The hens run free and have a more enjoyable life to produce healthier and tastier eggs.

Conjugated linoleic acid (CLA) is a natural polyunsaturated fatty acid found in many foods, including milk, cheese, and meats. The meat richest in CLA is beef, but it is also found in lamb and veal and, to a lesser degree, in pork, chicken, and turkey. CLA is made in the bellies of ruminants such as cows from grain fermented with the help of certain bacteria. In a study of CLA content under various feeding regimens, cows allowed to graze freely on the range had five hundred percent more CLA in their milkfat than cows fed typical dairy diets supplemented with corn silage or corn oil. CLA concentration is also increased when meats are cooked.

Evidence compiled over the last decade has led to the recognition that CLA possesses unique and potent antioxidant, anticarcinogenic (anticancer), and anticatabloic (helping to prevent metabolic destructiveness) effects. It is taken up by the body's phospholipids, a class of fats that serves as the principal structural components of cell membranes. CLA is now thought to represent a previously unidentified defense mechanism against membrane attack by oxygen radicals. It is also thought to help protect against atherosclerosis and cancer. It enhances body composition by helping increase muscle while reducing fat. Moreover, in animal studies, CLA has been shown to increase bone mass and exert a positive effect on diabetes by increasing insulin sensitivity.

CLA is produced synthetically by heating linoleic acid (an essential nutrient found widely in plant oils and animal fats) in the presence of a base. CLA increases HDL cholesterol and decreases LDL and triglycerides. It also enhances the immune system. CLA modulates leukotrienes and also suppresses the immunoglobin associated with allergies.

Although one can obtain neutral CLA from seared meats and milk, I recommend synthetic sources (see page 99). The seared meats may have a carcinogenic effect. Homogenized milk may work adversely in producing atherosclerosis secondary to xanthine oxidase (see page 290). CLA comes in 1000 mg doses taken daily and costs about a dollar a capsule. This is very safe and doses of 4000 mg a day are used to increase muscle and improve the immune function. The usual dose, though, is 1000 mg a day.

Monounsaturated fats (monos), are considered neutral, but many have some other effects, according to a 1999 article in the journal *Neurology* (52: 1563-1569). These oils, (olive oil in this case) decreased age related cognitive decline or Alzheimer's disease. Compared to other vegetable oils (the polyunsaturates) the monos have no adverse effect on the lipid profile. The oil with the most monos is canola (rapeseed), but the most commonly used is olive. Cold pressed extra-virgin oil is far better than other refined olive oils. Walnut oil has recently been shown to have better health properties. These oils have a higher content of alpha tocopheral and polyphenols. Compared to other processes of refinement they reduce the susceptibility of LDL cholesterol to oxidation and vascular uptake (atherosclerosis).

The cocoa in chocolate, especially dark chocolate, contains oligomeric proanthocyanidin (OPC), an active antioxidant compound. A recent study by a Harvard researcher, I. Min Lee, M.D. Sc.D., found that this candy is associated with an increased life span. Occasional indulgence in chocolate, or any fat for that matter, certainly makes life and eating more enjoyable. Though fats, even the good ones, are highly caloric, they are not categorically bad. In the right amounts they can prolong and enhance our well-being.

---

**Table 3-IV**
**FATTY ACIDS**

**Omega 3 series** — Alpha Linolenic Acid, Eicosstrienoic Acid, Eicosapentaenoic Acid, Docosahexaenoic Acid

**Omega 6 series** — Linoleic Acid, Gamma Linolenic Acid, Eicosadienoic Acid, Dihomo-Gammalinoleic Acid, Arachidonic Acid, Docosatetranoic Acid

**Omega 9 series** — Trans Elaidic Acid, Dis Oleic Acid Eicosenoic Acid, Euricic Acid, Nervonic Acid

**Saturated** — Palmitic Acid, Stearic Acid

---

## Cholesterol Reducers

The best thing since sliced bread could be the spreads invented to slather on it. Johnson & Johnson's *Benecol* and Lipton's *Take Control* are "nutraceuticals" or "functional foods" for customers who want what they eat to be therapeutic as well as tasty. They have beer available in the grocers since early 1999.

The key ingredients are plant sterols, which mimic the chemical structure of cholesterol and trick the digestive system into absorbing less of the real stuff. *(Benecol's* sterols are derived from pine wood pulp, *Take Control's* from soybeans.) The result is decreased production of LDL or "bad cholesterol." Clinical studies of *Benecol,* which has been sold without adverse effects in Finland since 1995, have shown that about one and a half tablespoons a day cut LDL cholesterol by ten to fourteen percent on average. A similar serving of *Take Control* produces a seven to ten percent reduction, according to Lipton. Paired with a diet low in saturated fats, the spreads can help reduce the LDL level up to twenty-five percent, or half as much as the drug simvastatin (Zocor™), some researchers say. To get the maximum benefit, you must eat the recommended portions of the spreads every day. Each product is available in pre-measured tubs as well as in bulk to help do that.

A panel of taste testers sampled *Benecol,* its lower-fat and -calorie version *Benecol Light, Take Control,* and other spreads containing a similar percentage of vegetable oil. They found that the plant-sterol spreads did not taste notably different than the others. The testers did note that the two *Benecol* spreads had a waxy, Crisco-like texture. On warm toast, *Benecol* behaved more like regular margarine than the others, though it never completely melted. *Benecol Light* did not melt; the *Take Control* toast turned damp and soggy. Note, too, that *Benecol* can be used in cooking and baking; *Take Control* and *Benecol Light* can't.

These are much less expensive than their prescription counterparts and in many cases as effective. Some evidence suggests that the active ingredient in Saw Palmetto, the herb used to prevent and treat prostate disease, is B-sitosterol, and a similar chemical to B-sitostanol. Saw Palmetto is fast gaining status in the U.S. as being equal to the very expensive prescription drug for prostate problems, Proscar®. These food products may be almost as good as saw palmetto for the prostate.

## Table 3-V
## Comparison of B-Sitostanol Products
## for Cholesterol and Possible Prostate Reduction

| | Serving Size and Active Ingredient | Mfr's Suggested Use | Retail Cost | Calories per Serving | Total Fat % Daily Value from Fat |
|---|---|---|---|---|---|
| Benecol® Spread (McNeil) | 1.5 tsp. (1.5g sitostanol) | a pat tid*** | $4.99 21 servings | 45 | 5 g/14% |
| Take Control™ Spread (Lipton) | 1 tbsp (1.12 g sitosterol) | 1 tbsp qd* | $3.79/ 21 servings | 50 | 6 g/9% |
| Benecol Light | 1 tbsp (1.5g sitosterol ester) | 1 pat tid*** | $4.99 8 oz. | 30 | 3 g/5% |
| Benecol® Ranch Salad Dressing** | 2 tbsp (1.5g sitostanol) | 2 tbsp* | $4.99/ 8 oz. | 130 | 13 g/20% |
| Take Control™ Reduced Fat Italian, Blue Cheese, Ranch Dressing** | 2 tbsp (1.12 g sitosterol) | 2 tbsp* | $3.79 8 oz. | 100 | 8 g/13% |

*daily        ** hard to obtain        ***thrice daily

## More about Cholesterol and other Lipids
In general, the higher our cholesterol, the more likely we are to have cardiovascular disease. The total cholesterol, however, is offset by the good cholesterol. That is, the HDL (high density lipoprotein) cholesterol is good; the LDL (low density lipoprotein) is bad. The total cholesterol is composed of the HDL (healing) cholesterol, the LDL (lousy) cholesterol and VLDL cholesterol. This seldom mentioned VLDL (very low density lipoprotein) cholesterol is a reflection of another fat, triglyceride, in our blood. Total cholesterol should be less than two hundred; LDL less than one hundred twenty-five. With high-risk patients the LDL is lowered to less than one

hundred. In extreme cases it is lowered to fifty. We only need twenty-five to survive. Of course, in order to lower the cholesterol like this drugs are needed.

Many doctors use a ratio of the total to the HDL cholesterol. The normal ratio is four. For every point above that there is a sixteen percent higher risk and conversely of having a cardiovascular event in the next five years. If our total cholesterol is two hundred, and our HDL is fifty, we have a ratio of four. Triglycerides should also be less than two hundred, according to some authorities, and still others say less than fifty! Unlike cholesterol, triglycerides fluctuate throughout the day; they are elevated when people eat. Thus, some doctors do a triglyceride tolerance test by giving patients a fatty meal, then two hours later a blood test. At this point, triglycerides over three hundred are detrimental to the blood vessels. Interestingly, in most individuals it is not what we eat, but how our body metabolizes our food that counts. In other words, the way our bodies handle lipids, or make fat, is under genetic control. In general, carbohydrates raise the triglycerides over the long run.

## II. PROTEIN

Protein is important because it provides amino acids, the building blocks for all mammalian tissue. It stimulates glucagon, a wonderful hormone from our pancreas. Every day our bodies use and lose protein. Unlike fats and carbohydrates, protein from any source is protein, although some have more essential amino acids and may have a better balance of these amino acids. Essential amino acids are those that our bodies can't produce, while nonessential amino acids are produced from any available protein.

Glucagon has the opposite action of insulin. It minimizes the adverse effects of too much insulin, which tend to make us fatter. The sources of all protein are fish, fowl, vegetables (legumes, whole grains), and red meats. Non-animal sources are better than animal sources in that the methionine of the latter is converted in the body to homocysteine, which has been shown for the last three decades to be a significant risk factor in cardiocerebral disease. Books like *Protein Power*, a best-seller several years ago, by Dr. Michael and Mary Eads have indoctrinated many Americans into the consumption of lots of protein.

| Table 3-VI<br>Foods with lots of protein | |
|---|---|
| Half a cup of cottage cheese | 16 grams |
| One cup of yogurt | 12 grams |
| Half a cup of tofu | 10 grams |
| Half a cup of kidney beans | 8 grams |
| One ounce of nuts | 6 grams |

There is a down-side in consuming too much protein. If one has diabetes and kidney disease, it can elevate the protein in the urine, making the kidneys fail faster. It has also been shown to cause osteoporosis. There are no problems, however, if eaten in the proper amounts; I suggest thirty percent. Plant sources are my first choice, and fish, second.

**Vegetable** protein, like all non-animal foods, has no cholesterol. Vegetables are also a good source of fiber, vitamins, and minerals. They can, however, contain a fair amount of carbohydrates. It is better to eat the leaves (lettuce, spinach), flowers (broccoli, cauliflower), and stems (asparagus, celery) than the fruits (plums, tomatoes) or, worse, the roots (potatoes, carrots), in order to limit carbohydrates. Legumes such as chick peas or beans are also good sources of protein, as is soy, which will be discussed later.

**Fish** protein is rich in Omega 3 fatty acids (EPA and DHA). Fat from any source is calorie-dense, but this kind, at least, is full of healthy properties.

**Fowl** is also a good choice of protein, and the white meat has less fat than the dark. As in all animal sources of protein, there is some non-harmful cholesterol, too.

**Red meats,** including beef, pork, and lamb, have protein, but the meat should be lean. Meat fat is saturated, which is not good for the cardiovascular system. It is also highly caloric. We do not need to be concerned about the cholesterol in meat, but we should be aware of the remote possibility of pesticide and antibiotic accumulation. Both of these are concentrated in the fat, which we should avoid anyway. The more the meat is cooked, the more fat is removed. Grilling it or placing it on a porous tray will help the fat drip out. Meat is an excellent source of many minerals such as iron, zinc, and magnesium, and it does contain some vitamins. Organ meats such as liver should be eaten minimally or not at all since they contain a lot of fat. Burning of fats not only oxidizes them, causing more free radicals, but is also carcinogenic.

## The Joy of Soy

Soy used to be degraded as a food impostor, an illegitimate filler, but now its healthiness and versatility have transformed its reputation. It is a complete protein like meat, milk, and eggs. It is also a low insulin producer, glycemic index of twenty-five, and a preventer of vascular disease and cancer. A recent article intimated that replacing half the meat in our diet with a different source of protein will increase life expectancy by thirteen percent (about ten years). Soy also has specific medical benefits. Two of its isoflavones, Genistein and Diazosin, are estrogen substitutes. Major studies have shown that they adhere to the estrogen receptors in the breasts, uterus, and even the brain. As such, they prevent the foreign estrogens (Xenoestrogens) of agricultural contaminants like pesticides from adhering to these tissues and inducing cancer in susceptible patients. Some women who take soy or its specific isoflavones in the appropriate amounts have no need to take estrogen. Soy also has an affinity for the beta-receptor, which is the most important of all the estrogen receptors. The brain has this receptor, while other tissues, including blood vessels, breast, and uterus, have both alpha and beta receptors.

Soy can be eaten as a nut, lightly salted and seasoned

with spices. Commercial companies sell this, or we can buy soybeans for only pennies a pound and make our own. Soy comes in many other forms as well. Tempeh is a cultured soybean made into a dense loaf. Tofu is a versatile curd that can be firm or soft. TVP (Texturized Vegetable Protein) is another soy product that comes in granules which can be used as chopped meat (Hamburger Helper is made up almost entirely of TVP) or in chunks which can be used in stew. The advantage of TVP is that it has absolutely no taste of its own, so it takes on the ambiance of whatever sauce or spice is used with it. I recall a barbecue cook-off in a small western town where, as a gag, an individual used TVP chunks with K.C. Masterpiece Barbecue Sauce. The concoction won first prize! We may want to keep children and husbands out of the kitchen when we work with TVP because it looks like dog food. TVP can be purchased in some supermarkets, health food stores, or through mail-order houses. It is not expensive and is very healthy. Soy is also commercially incorporated into pizza, cheesecake, and healthy snacks. Recently, there have been some negative press regarding soy. The denaturing of the soy protein as found in TVP makes our body think it is a foreign protein and is not used as well. Whole soybeans, per se, are not nearly as digestible as the fermentation soy products. Please see Table 3-VII, pages 84 and 85 for the variety of soy food products available.

## III. CARBOHYDRATES

Carbohydrates are sugar and starch found in vegetables, grain (starch), fruit (simple sugars), legumes, milk (disaccharides), and in refined sugars and flour. They should be consumed in moderation because carbohydrates stimulate insulin production from the pancreas. There is a direct correlation between how much and how quickly carbohydrates are eaten and how much insulin is released. Insulin itself is not bad, but it is dangerous in excess amounts. It elevates blood pressure, causes atherosclerosis, produces bad eicosanoids (a type of hormone), decreases the ability to concentrate, and

# TABLE 3-VII

## THE INCREDIBLE EDIBLE SOY

**Green Vegetable — Soybeans (Edamame)** These large soybeans are harvested when the beans are still green and sweet tasting and can be served as a snack or a main vegetable dish, after boiling in slightly salted water after 15-20 minutes. They are high in protein and fiber and contain no cholesterol.

**Texturized Vegetable Protein (TVP) —** Texturized vegetable protein (TVP) is a protein obtained from any vegetable, including soybeans. The protein is broken down into amino acids by a chemical process called acid hydrolysis. HVP is a flavor enhancer that can be used in soups, broths, sauces, gravies, flavoring and spice blends. See textured soy protein and flour, page 85.

**Meat Alternatives (Meat Analogs) —** Meat alternatives made from soybeans contain soy protein or tofu and other ingredients mixed together to simulate various kinds of meat. These meat alternatives are sold as frozen, canned or dried foods. Usually, they can be used the same way as the foods they replace. With so many different meat alternatives available to consumers, the nutritional value of these foods varies considerably. Generally, they are lower in fat, but read the label to be certain. Meat alternatives made from soybeans are excellent sources of protein, iron and B vitamins.

**Miso —** Miso is a rich, salty condiment that characterizes the essence of Japanese cooking. The Japanese make miso soup and use it to flavor a variety of foods. A smooth paste, miso is made from soybeans and a grain such as rice, plus salt and a mold culture, and then aged in cedar vats for one to three years. Miso should be refrigerated. Use miso to flavor soups, sauces, dressings, marinades and pates.

**Natto —** Natto is made of fermented, cooked whole soybeans. Because the fermentation process breaks down the beans' complex proteins, natto is more easily digested than whole soybeans. It has a sticky, viscous coating with a cheesy texture. In Asian countries natto traditionally is served as a topping for rice, in miso soups and is used with vegetables. Natto can be found in Asian natural food stores.

**Non-dairy Soy Frozen Desserts —** Non-dairy frozen desserts are made from soymilk or soy yogurt. Soy ice cream is one of the most popular desserts made from soybeans.

**Soy Cheese —** Soy cheese is made from soymilk. Its creamy texture makes it an easy substitute for most cheeses, sour cream or cream cheese and can be found in a variety of flavors. Products made with soy cheese include soy pizza.

**Soy Fiber (Okara, Soy Bran, Soy Isolate Fiber) —** There are three basic types of soy fiber: okara, soy bran and soy isolate fiber. All of these products are high-quality, inexpensive sources of dietary fiber.

**Okara** is a pulp fiber by-product of soymilk. It has less protein than whole soybeans, but the protein remaining is of high quality. Okara tastes similar to coconut and can be baked or added as fiber to granola and cookies. Okara also has been made into sausage.

**Soy bran** is made from hulls (the outer covering of the soybean) which are removed during initial processing. The hulls contain a fibrous material which can be extracted and then refined for use as a food ingredient.

**Soy isolate fiber,** also known as structured protein fiber (SPF), is soy protein isolate in a fibrous form.

**Soy Flour —** Soy flour is made from roasted soybeans ground into a fine powder. There are three kinds of soy flour available:
• Natural or full-fat, which contains the natural oils found in the soybean;
• Defatted, which has the oils removed during processing;
• Lecithinated, which has had lecithin added to it.

All soy flour gives a protein boost to recipes. However, defatted soy flour is an even more concentrated source of protein than full-fat soy flour. Soy flour is gluten-free, so yeast-raised breads made with soy flour are more dense in texture.

**Soy Grits —** Soy grits are similar to soy flour except that the soybeans have been toasted and cracked into coarse pieces, rather than the fine powder of soy flour. Soy grits can be used as a substitute for flour in some recipes. High in protein, soy grits can be added to rice and other grains and cooked together.

**Soy Protein Concentrate —** Soy protein concentrate comes from defatted soy flakes. It contains about 70 percent protein, while retaining most of the bran's dietary fiber.

**Soy Protein Isolate (Isolated Soy Protein) —** When protein is removed from defatted flakes, the result is soy protein isolate, the most highly refined soy protein. Containing 92 percent protein, soy protein isolates possess the greatest amount of protein of all soy products. They are a highly digestible source of amino acids (building blocks of protein necessary for human growth and maintenance.

**Soy Protein, Textured** — Textured soy protein (TSP) usually refers to products made from textured soy flour, although the term can also be applied to textured soy protein concentrates and spun soy fiber.

**Textured soy flour** (TSF) is made by running defatted soy flour through an extrusion cooker, which allows for many different forms and sizes. When hydrated, it has a chewy texture. It is widely used as a meat extender. Textured soy flour contains about 70 percent protein and retains most of the bean's dietary fiber. Often referred to simply as textured soy protein (TSP), textured soy flour is sold dried in granular and chunk style.

**Soy Sauce** — (Tamari, Shoyu, Teriyaki) Soy sauce is a dark brown liquid made from soybeans that have undergone a fermenting process. Soy sauces have a salty taste, but are lower in sodium than traditional table salt. Specific types of soy sauce are: shoyu, tamari and teriyaki. Shoyu is a blend of soybeans and what. Tamari is made only from soybeans and is a by-product of making miso. Teriyaki sauce can be thicker than other types of soy sauce and includes other ingredients such as sugar, vinegar and spices.

**Soy Yogurt** — Soy yogurt is made from soymilk. Its creamy texture makes it an easy substitute for sour cream or cream cheese. Soy yogurt can be found in variety of flavors in natural food stores.

**Soybeans** — As soybeans mature in the pods, they ripen into a hard, dry bean. Although most soybeans are yellow, there also are brown and black varieties. Whole soybeans (an excellent source of protein and dietary fiber) can be cooked and used in sauces, stews and soups. Whole soybeans that have been soaked can be roasted for snacks. When grown without agricultural chemicals, they are referred to as organically grown soybeans.

**Soymilk, Soy Beverages** —Soybeans, soaked, ground fine and strained, produce a fluid called soybean milk which is a good substitute for cow's milk. Plain, unfortified soymilk is an excellent source of high quality protein and B-vitamins. Soymilk is most commonly found in aseptic containers (non-refrigerated, shelf stable), but also can be found in quart and half-gallon containers in the dairy case at the supermarket. Soymilk is also sold as a powder which must be mixed with water.

**Soynut Butter** — Made from roasted, whole soynuts, which are then crushed and blended with soybean oil and other ingredients. Soynut butter has a slightly nutty taste, significantly less fat than peanut butter and provides many other nutritional benefits as well.

**Soynuts** — Roasted soynuts are whole soybeans that have been soaked in water and then baked until browned. Soynuts can be found in a variety of flavors, including chocolate-covered. High in protein and isoflavones, soynuts are similar in texture and flavor to peanuts.

**Sprouts, Soy** — Although not as popular as mung bean sprouts or alfalfa sprouts, soy sprouts (also called soybean sprouts), are an excellent source of nutrition, packed with protein and vitamin C.

**Tempeh** — Tempeh, a traditional Indonesian food, is a chunky, tender soybean cake. Whole soybeans, sometimes mixed with another grain such as rice or millet, are fermented into a rich cake of soybeans with a smoky or nutty flavor. Tempeh can be marinated and grilled and added to soups, casseroles or chili.

**Tofu and Tofu Products** — Tofu, also known as soybean curd, is a soft, cheese-like food made by curdling fresh hot soymilk with a coagulant. Tofu is a bland product that easily absorbs the flavors of other ingredients with which it is cooked. Tofu is rich in high-quality protein, B-vitamins and low in sodium. Firm tofu is dense and solid and can be cubed and served in soups, stir-fried or grilled. Firm tofu is higher in protein, fat and calcium than other forms of tofu. Soft tofu is good for recipes that call for blended tofu. Silken tofu is a creamy product and can be used as a replacement for sour cream in many dip recipes.

**Whipped Toppings, Soy-Based** — Soy-based whipped toppings are similar to other non-dairy whipped toppings, except that hydrogenated soybean oil is used instead of other vegetable oils.

**Yuba** — Yuba is made by lifting and drying the thin layer formed on the surface of cooling hot soymilk. It has a high protein content and is commonly sold fresh, half-dried and dried. In the U.S., dried yuba sheets (called dried bean curd, bean curd sheets, or bean curd skin) and u-shaped rolls (called bamboo yuba or bean curd sticks) can be found in Asian food stores.

makes us fat by making us feel hungry and placing our most recent food consumption directly into our fat cells. Most adult onset diabetics produce too much insulin.

Glucagon, another hormone produced by the pancreas mainly when we eat protein, neutralizes the adverse effect of insulin. Thus, it is important to eat as much protein as carbohydrates. Some nutritionists recommend eating protein before eating carbohydrates. Excess carbohydrate consumption causes water production and, at times, water retention, since these are metabolized to carbon dioxide and water.

One needs to consider the total amount of calories, as well as the glycemic index (see later) in that if one eats caloric dense foods such as fat, it certainly will add to our already fattened bodies. With extra insulin, fat goes right into the fat cell; whereas if carbohydrates change to fat, it has a metabolic cost of only 23% and less calories go to fat. The lower the **GLYCEMIC INDEX (GI)**, the healthier.

The glycemic index (GI) was first developed in 1981 by a team of scientists led by Dr. David Jenkins, then at the University of Toronto to help determine which foods were best for folks with diabetes. At that time, the diet for diabetics was based on a system of carbohydrate exchanges. It was so complex, it was not easily taught to patients.

The American Diabetic Association did not accept the GI concept, but is now coming to the conclusion that it is important in the fare of a diabetic. In an article in September, 2000 *American Journal of Clinical Nutrition*, eating low on the GI enhances memory and cognition, as well as help weight loss, lowering blood sugar, enhancing energy and preventing vascular disease. Much more work was done at The University of Sydney in Australia four years ago. A book called *The GI Factor* authored by Jennie Brand-Miller, Ph.D. was published in 1996. It wasn't until recently that this book came out in the U.S. in paperback published by Marlow and Company for $14.95 titled *The Glucose Revolution*.

It is a physiologic fact that only glucose stimulates pancreatic insulin release. The faster and the higher glucose is released in digestion, the more the insulin in the blood. In-

# Table 3-VIII
## GLYCEMIC INDEX

The higher the Glycemic Index, the more insulin the food will produce. Eating foods lower on the Glycemic Index will encourage weight loss by lowering the insulin level.

## High Inducers of Insulin (Bad)

**Grain-based foods (GI>100)**
Puffed rice
Corn flakes
Puffed wheat
Millet
Instant rice
Instant potatoes
Microwave popcorn
French bread
**Simple Sugars**
Maltose
Glucose

**Grain based foods (GI 80-100)**
Grapenuts
Whole-wheat bread
Rolled oats
Oat bran
White bread
Instant mashed
 potatoes
White rice
Brown rice
Muesli
Shredded wheat

**Vegetables**
Carrots
Parsnips
Corn
**Fruits**
Bananas
Raisins
Apricots
Papaya
Mango
**Snacks**
Tofu ice cream
Puffed rice cakes
Ice cream
Corn chips
Rice crisps

## Moderate Inducers of Insulin (Better)

**Grain-based foods (GI>50-80)**
Spaghetti (white)
Spaghetti (whole wheat)
Pasta, other
Pumpernickel bread
All-bran cereal

**Fruits**
Orange
Orange juice
**Vegetables**
Peas
Pinto beans
Garbanzo beans
Kidney beans
Baked beans

**Simple sugars**
Lactose
Sucrose
**Snacks**
Candy bars
Potato chips (with fat)

## Reduced Insulin Secretors (Good)

**Grain-based foods (GI 30-50)**
Barley
Oatmeal
 (slow cooking)
Whole-grain rye bread
**Fruits**
Apples
Apple juice

Applesauce
Pears
Grapes
Peaches
**Vegetables**
Peas
Lentils
Black-eyed peas
Chick-peas

Kidney beans (dried)
Lima beans
Tomato soup
**Dairy products**
Yogurt
Ice cream (high fat)
Milk (skim)
Milk (whole)

## Lowest Insulin Inducers (Best)

**Fruits (GI <30)**
Cherries
Plums
Grapefruit

**Simple sugars**
Fructose
**Vegetables**
Soy beans

**Snacks**
peanuts

# Table 3-IX
## GLYCEMIC INDEX ACCORDING TO NUMBERS

Not all carbohydrates are created equal. They cause our pancreas to make insulin, which causes weight gain, arteriosclerosis, high blood pressure and poor health. The lower on the GI index, the less insulin is produced.

**FOOD**        **GI INDEX**

**BREAKFAST CEREALS**
- Kellogg's All-Bran w/extra fiber® ..... 51
- Kellogg's Corn Flakes® ...................... 84
- Kellogg's Raisin Bran® ...................... 73
- Kellogg's Rice Krispies® ................... 82
- Kellogg's Special K® .......................... 54
- Oatmeal (old fashioned) ................... 49
- Post Shredded Wheat® ...................... 57

**GRAINS/PASTAS**
- Bulgur ................................................. 48
- Rice
  - Basmati ......................................... 58
  - brown ............................................. 55
  - long grain, white ........................... 56
  - short grain, white ......................... 72
  - Uncle Ben's Converted® ............... 44
  - parboiled ........................................ 48
- Noodles—instant ................................ 46
- Spaghetti ............................................ 41

**BREADS, MUFFINS AND CAKES**
- Bagel .................................................. 72
- Croissant ............................................ 67
- Pita bread .......................................... 57
- Pumpernickel (whole grain) .............. 51
- Rye bread ........................................... 76
- Sourdough bread ................................ 52
- Sponge cake ....................................... 46
- Stoneground whole wheat ................. 53
- Waffles ................................................ 76
- White bread ........................................ 70
- Whole wheat bread ............................ 69

**CRACKERS/CRISPBREAD**
- Water cracker ..................................... 78

**COOKIES**
- Graham crackers ................................ 74
- Oatmeal .............................................. 55
- Vanilla Wafers ................................... 77

**VEGETABLES**
- Beets ................................................... 64
- Carrots ................................................ 49
- Parsnip ............................................... 97
- Peas (green) ....................................... 48
- Potato
  - baked .............................................. 93
  - new ................................................. 62
  - red-skinned .................................... 88
  - French fries .................................... 75
- Pumpkin .............................................. 75
- Sweet corn .......................................... 55
- Sweet potato ....................................... 54

**LEGUMES**
- Baked beans ....................................... 48
- Broad beans ........................................ 79
- Butter beans ....................................... 31
- Chick peas .......................................... 33
- Kidney beans ...................................... 27
- Lentils ................................................. 30

**FOOD**        **GI INDEX**

- Navy beans .......................................... 38
- Soy beans ............................................ 18
- Chana dal ............................................. 8

**FRUIT**
- Apple ................................................... 38
- Apricot (dried) ................................... 31
- Banana ................................................ 55
- Cantaloupe ......................................... 65
- Cherries .............................................. 22
- Dates, dried ..................................... 103
- Grapefruit ........................................... 25
- Grapes ................................................. 46
- Kiwi ..................................................... 52
- Orange ................................................ 44
- Papaya ................................................ 58
- Pear ..................................................... 38
- Pineapple ............................................ 66
- Plum .................................................... 39
- Raisins ................................................ 64
- Watermelon ........................................ 72

**DAIRY FOODS**
- Milk
  - whole .............................................. 27
  - skim ................................................ 32
  - chocolate flavored ......................... 34
- Ice cream ............................................ 61
  - low fat ............................................ 50
- Yogurt, flavored, low fat ................... 33

**BEVERAGES**
- Apple juice ......................................... 40
- Flavored syrup (diluted) ................... 66
- Fanta® ................................................ 68
- Gatorade® ........................................... 78
- Orange juice ....................................... 46

**SNACK FOODS**
- Corn chips .......................................... 72
- Peanuts ............................................... 14
- Popcorn ............................................... 55
- Potato chips ........................................ 54
- Pretzels ............................................... 83
- Power Bar® Performance ................... 58

**CANDY**
- Chocolate ............................................ 49
- Jelly beans .......................................... 80
- Life Savers® ....................................... 70
- Mars Almond Bars ............................. 68
- Twix Cookie Bar® .............................. 44
- Snickers® ........................................... 41
- Skittles Fruit Chews® ....................... 70

**SUGARS**
- Fructose .............................................. 23
- Glucose .............................................. 100
- Honey .................................................. 58
- Lactose ................................................ 46
- Maltose .............................................. 105
- Sucrose ............................................... 65

sulin is a two-edged sword. The good is needed to drive sugar into the cells, but if too much glucose (and subsequently, too much insulin) is in our system it can have a damaging effect, causing high blood pressure, adverse lipids, increase of arteriosclerosis and worst of all to our vanity, *obesity*. Food is energy, but if that energy cannot be used immediately, it is initially stored as glycogen in the liver and subsequently, into the adipose cell as *fat*.

Food is ranked on a scale from 0 to 100, with glucose having the index of 100. The higher the index, the more insulin is released from the pancreas and the more fat is produced to be stored. Table sugar (sucrose) has a GI of 65 . Fructose alone has a GI of only 23. Starches have the highest GI, with a potato having 101! On the other hand, white bread has 72, stone ground whole wheat has 53. Pastas are not nearly as bad, with spaghetti having a GI of only 41. White rice has a GI of 72, but Uncle Ben's Converted Rice is 44. Dried dates are 103, apples 38, oranges 44, grapefruit 25 and cherries 22. The less ripe the fruit, the better. Green-yellow rather than brown-yellow bananas and Granny Smith green apples are better than red. Parboiling or not overcooking decreases the GI. The starch, which is stored in a protein packet and is broken by cooking, increasing the GI. Thus al dente pasta(firm to the bite) will have a lower GI. A fantastic tasty and filling grain that is tasty and filling is barley with a GI of 25. China dal (a legume) is only 8.

Low GI foods are filling. Eating slowly physically lowers the glycemic index in that the food goes into the intestines less rapidly with less production of insulin. Taking lemon juice or vinegar will tend to lower the GI of all foods. These acids decrease the stomach emptying rate. Adding lemon juice or vinegar to part of the salad dressing works well. Consuming a mixture of high and low glycemic index together result in an intermediate GI. Frequent small meals are better than large meals, breakfast being the most important. Therefore, skipping meals until a late supper is bad for the body's economy of active (kinetic) energy, but does give potential energy, which of course is fat.

# The Mushroom Boon

Mushrooms have been favored for centuries, not only as food, but also as remedies against aging. I will mention three of them: the Reishi, the Shiitake, and the Maitake. According to some practitioners, the Reishi has been used clinically against cancer, cardiovascular disease, chronic fatigue syndrome, hepatitis, herpes, hypertension, high cholesterol, HIV, and for weight loss. The Shiitake, a first cousin to the Reishi and Japan's largest agricultural export, has been used as a remedy for upper respiratory disease, poor circulation, and fatigue. It may also prevent premature aging. Today, however, it is recognized most for its immunologic activity and as an anti-tumor agent. The Maitaki, also from Japan, has been advocated to strengthen the body and improve overall health. These are giant mushrooms, often twenty inches in diameter; a single cluster can weigh up to one hundred pounds. Recently they have also been used against hepatitis, cancer, HIV, and for regulating blood pressure and blood sugar. Aside from the medical benefits, mushrooms taste good, are low in calories, very filling, and not too costly.

# Fiber

Fiber is important because it cleans our digestive system like a good scrub brush and diminishes such diseases as cancer, diabetes, diverticuloses(itis), gall stones, hemorrhoids, and even appendicitis. Regarding cancer, its preventative effectiveness is unclear. A recent study shows that fiber did not have any effect on colon cancer. According to the 1999 *American Journal of Gastroenerology*, it is low animal product consumption that is beneficial, not fiber. The method of defecation is also preventive of these gastrointestinal diseases than the type and fiber content of food. Going only when necessary and squatting over, rather than sitting on, a toilet with three-inch blocks under the feet and squeezing the upper calves is recommended. Fiber can be soluble or insoluble. It is a non-absorbable carbohydrate and therefore contributes no calories.

## Phytochemicals

Phyto is a Greek root meaning "plants." Thus, the buzz word, "phytochemical," refers to a chemical of plant origin. Every year science discovers more of these and their numerous sub-types. For example, lycopene, which is found in tomatoes, and in even higher amounts in processed tomato products like spaghetti and pizza sauce. This not only discourages tumor growth, particularly in the prostate, but it also protects the eyes. See Table 3-X , page 94, for foods containing other phytochemicals and their properties.

## Fire in the Hole

One could classify hot sauce, the spicy kind, not the elevated temperature of a heated sauce, as a food or herb, but we will discuss this under food because the main ingredient is the pepper. Since the days of Columbus, peppers have been used to flavor and preserve both meats and vegetables: the hotter the pepper, the less bacteria will grow. The heat in peppers is measured scientifically in Scoville Heat Units. Wilkes Scoville was a pharmacologist who, in 1912, developed the method of quantifying the "heat" in a pepper. The mildest bell pepper has zero units, sometimes referred to as heat units or H.U., while habaneros rate three hundred thousand units. Incidentally, mace has only two hundred thousand units, my son, a police officer, told me. Even a mild bell pepper grown twenty yards away from a cayenne can claim some Scoville Heat potential. The hottest are chipotle regula and the habanero (Scotchbonnet pepper).

The active ingredient in hot peppers is *capsaicin* (see Table 3-X, page 94), which, as many arthritis sufferers know, can be rubbed on an inflamed joint with much relief; although, the first time or two, it will burn the skin. Capsaicin antagonizes the action of substance P, the neurotransmitter or chemical that activates the neuron (nerve cell) that transfers the message from a pain site to the brain. In addition to blocking pain, Capsaicin stimulates circulation, aids digestion, and, as those of us who have used hot peppers know, promotes sweating. Because perspiration works to cool the body, cayenne is sometimes used to break a fever. Post operative pain, cluster headaches, shingles, and aching skin are other occasions to use capsaicin.

An occasion, however, is hardly necessary. Tobasco sauce has been around since 1868, when the McIlhenny family of Louisiana developed the formula. Today it is a standard condiment in most homes and restaurants. Similarly, salsa is now served to schoolchildren who also eat tobasco flavored jelly beans. Considered by some as simply flavor enhancers or salt substitutes, these sauces have also been credited with decongesting nasal passages, boosting the metabolism, enhancing the immune system, and even extending life. In addition to the hot peppers, these sauces may include other ingredients such as vinegar, salt, or mustard seeds. If the sauce has fruits or vegetables in it, refrigerate after opening, unless it will be consumed within a month. Unfortunately, the sauces are not rated according to Scoville Heat Units but with the subjective descriptors mild, medium hot, and hot. There are many variations of each, but the names may provide a clue: "Cape Fear," "Hellter and Damnation," "Capital Punishment" and "Screaming Sphincter." All, especially the last, warn of fire in the hole. Contrary to popular belief, these fiery peppers themselves do not cause ulcers, although some folks may be intolerant and/or unaccustomed to their spiciness. Most problems come instead from the food on which the sauce is placed. Antidotes for the heat, at least, include yogurt and other dairy products.

**Fruits**

Fruits are another cancer and age fighting food. Strawberries, blueberries and, the best, the English bilberry, are all high in antioxidants. I also suggest eating grapefruit or drinking the juice daily. It makes certain drugs, such as statins (for lowering cholesterol), calcium antagonists, ACE inhibitors (anti-hypertensives), digoxin, and non-steroidal anti-inflammatory drugs somewhat more powerful by increasing their activation. Grapefruit has a Glycemic Index of only thirty-six, and Naringenin, one of its active substances, may also speed up our metabolism. Similarly, its limonoid (see Table 3-X, page 94) helps the immune system detoxify carcinogenic compounds. One large grapefruit or a glass of juice may last the body all day. This might be why grapefruit is the cornerstone of the "Mayo Clinic Diet" for weight loss. The content of limonoid and naringenin varies among juice types and brands. Fresh ruby red grapefruit contains the most. One can discount the calories in this fruit since it increases caloric burnoff.

## Health is as Easy as A-B-C
## (Acidophilus-Bifido-Certified Live Active Yogurt)

Yogurt is low in calories and fat, but probiotics may be the real secret to its biggest health benefits. The live cultures in yogurt create its creamy texture and sour taste as well as a healthy intestine. These bacteria are called *probiotics,* a term that means "for life" and refers to any live organism in food that has benefits beyond simple nutrition. Probiotics are also showing up in all sorts of health food drinks and supplements, though yogurt is still their main source.

The two key bacteria in regular yogurt are *Streptococcus thermophilus* and *Lactobacillus bulgaricus.* Their work is to turn milk into yogurt by gorging on the milk's sugar, or lactose, and converting it to lactic acid. The lactic acid works the proteins into such knots that the whole solution curdles. This fermentation allows even people with lactose intolerance to eat this dairy product. Yogurt bacteria also contain their own lactase, which goes to work on any milk sugar that is left over from fermentation. When these bacteria hit the small intestine, digestive juices split them open, releasing enough lactase to break down the milk.

A variety of *Lactobacillus* called acidophilus and the latest, *Bifidobacterium* (or bifido), are added to the culture. Researchers have been aware of bifido since the early 1900s, but few strains survive well in yogurt. Unlike other bacteria, which are killed by stomach acids, these wade past the stomach and settle in the small and large intestines. They manage to thrive in the intestine's balanced ecosystem of

# Table 3-X
# PHYTOCHEMICALS:
## What they do and which foods have them?

| Phytochemical | Possible Action | Food Source |
|---|---|---|
| Allicin. allylic sulfides | Induce emcymatic detoxification systems; may act against *Helicobacter pylori;* allylic sulfides may reduce BP and cholesterol levels. | Onions, garlic, scallions, leeks chives |
| Capsaicin | Neutralizes carcinogenic benzopyrenes/substance P. | Chili peppers |
| Catichins | Reduce cholesterol levels preventing oxidation; inhibit phase I and II enzyme systems, which plays a role in carcinogen activation. | Green tea, straw berries, raspberries and other berries. |
| Chlorogenic acid | Blocks formation of carcinogenic nitrosamines | Tomatoes, green peppers,pineapples. |
| Flavonoids (4,000 different compounds, including flavonols, isoflavones, and flavones) | Antioxidants; reduce cell proliferation; increase the pump-mediated efflux of certain carcinogens from cells; isoflavones inhibit bone resorption. | Widely distributed in fruits, vegetables, wine, tea. |
| Indoles | Spur enzymes to form an estrogen; thought to be protective against breast, colon, esophageal, prostrate and lung cancers. | Cabbage, broccoli, Brussels sprouts, cauliflower, kale collards, mustard greens, turnips, rutabaga. |
| Limonoids | Increase production of protective enzymes | Citrus fruits, particularly the rind. |
| Monoterpenes | Antioxidants | Broccoli, cabbage, citrus fruits, cucumbers, eggplant, parsley, peppers, squash, tomatoes,yams. |
| P-Coumnaric acid | Blocks production of cancer-causing nitrosamines | Tomatoes, green peppers,pineapple, strawberries. |
| Protease inhibitors | Lengthen the time it takes for cancer cells to develop. | Soybeans, cereals, beans. |
| Triterenoids | Suppress carcinogenic activity of estrogen. | Soybeans, licorice root extract, citrus fruits, carrots |

other benign and beneficial bacteria.

When this equilibrium is upset by harmful food-borne bacteria, like salmonella or campylobacter, diarrhea frequently results. Acidophilus and bifido may help suppress such an infection by crowding spaces where damaging bacteria would otherwise attach themselves and by releasing acids that destroy the invading germs. Reseeding the intestine with these beneficial microbes can also stem the diarrhea and other side effects of some antibiotics. Since antibiotics are indiscriminate in their wrath, killing good bacteria along with the bad, at the end of a ten-day course a person may have a seriously depleted intestine. Eating yogurt along the way can control the damage.

Acidophilus yogurt may combat vaginal yeast infections as well. In a 1992 study of thirty-three women with recurrent infections, those who ate eight ounces of acidophilus-rich yogurt daily for six months had significantly fewer infections than in the previous six months. They also fared better than women who ate no yogurt at all.

Probiotics may also fuel the immune system in a more generalized way. A 1997 study showed that yogurt with acidophilus appeared to increase the activity of phagocytes, the white blood cells that destroy invading germs. Other studies suggest bifido might be a cancer fighter. A 1996 analysis showed that eating yogurt containing bifido bacteria switched off an enzyme associated with colon cancer.

Any yogurt that has at least one hundred million live bacteria per gram, the minimum believed necessary for health effects, carries the LAC (live active culture) seal. Products with the heavier-duty probiotics also list acidophilus and bifido. A-B yogurt is at this time hard to find in the U.S., but common in Europe and modern Asia. Even a few frozen yogurts meet the criteria. The yogurt is frozen so fast that the live cultures aren't destroyed; they are held in suspended animation, and once the yogurt thaws, the salutary microbes are revived. Bacteria aside, there are many other healthful reasons to eat yogurt. For one, it is a powerhouse of calcium, even better than a comparable serving of milk or cheese (see page 296).

It is relatively easy to make your own yogurt. Just buy a starter package from a health food store and follow the directions on the label, or ask a healthy friend to give you four ounces of his or her already prepared yogurt. You can also begin with a grocery store brand of live Acidophilus yogurt that is specifically labeled as such. Using a home yogurt maker with an automatic incubator is also a possibility. We bought ours from *The Old Country Store,* (501) 624-1248, for under fifty dollars. Each time we make yogurt we save four ounces with which to begin the next batch. I have known some families who brought their yogurt culture from Europe decades ago and still use it.

## Smarty Plants

Although the precise definition of the term "organically grown" is much debated, there is a growing consensus that these fruits and vegetables are healthier. The pesticides, herbicides, and fertilizers used in conventional growing do have a certain amount of toxicity that gradually takes its toll in human dysfunction and premature death. For example, in the journal *Lancet*, a study revealed that men who ate organic foods produced forty-three percent more sperm than those who do not. Unfortunately, isolating and eliminating these substances are tricky. A fertilizer that is otherwise all natural might, for instance, contain a cow patty that was treated with hormones and/or antibiotics while alive.

Genetic engineering of food plants is another controversial subject. The new breed of genetically modified tomatoes that hit the market in 1994 made a rotten splash in Europe. The safety of genetically altered food is still vociferously debated in the European common market and is starting to polarize this country.

These so-called "Frankenfoods" are actually more common than most people realize: fifty-five percent of soybeans and thirty-five percent of corn crops are genetically engineered. A growing array of fruits and vegetables comes from specially designed genes. In 1992 the FDA declared these man-made foods safe on the grounds that they were not significantly different than other crossbred varieties like nectarines (derived from peaches) and tangelos (from tangerines and grapefruit).

The green nay-sayers point out that previously foods were crossbred with related genes, within the same gene family. Frankenfoods, on the other hand, have no such limitation. Genes from essentially different organisms such as yeast, bacteria, or even animals are inserted into food plants. The possibilities are endless, unknown, and most important, may have a different vibration or spin compared to natural products.

The benefits, however, are as persuasive as the drawbacks. Plants are already engineered to be more resistant to cold weather and pests, and to require shorter growing seasons and less fertilizer. This same technology can also create nutritionally power-packed food plants: fruits and vegetables that deliver more vitamins; nuts, milk, and cereals that are allergy free; plant "toothbrushes" that contain a chemical to prevent decay; plant oils with more omega 3's; and food with increased macronutrients. These are referred to as functional foods.

So far congress has not required food producers to label genetically engineered products. Bill HR 3377, the Genetically Engineered Food Right to Know Act, which will be brought to the House by 2001, would require both the FDA and USPA to label all such food. So be it; there is no harm in labels. The real issue is public awareness.

## DRINKING

Three-fourths of modern humankind are dehydrated. A healthy lifestyle requires plenty of fluids. These should be in the form of natural water, mineral water, herbal teas, or, the best, grapefruit juice. Besides keeping the body running, simply quaffing enough has many specific benefits. Drinking eight ounces of liquid before a meal may help blunt the appetite. Furthermore, fat metabolism requires more water consumption than do carbohydrate and protein metabolism. Constipation can also be avoided by enough fluid consumption. Two quarts of fluids, mostly water, are recommended daily. Diet drinks containing artificial sweeteners are not recommended because they can stimulate the appetite, and some people (five percent) experience headaches, confusion, and rarely, even seizures with NutraSweet. If, however, we have no side effects, it doesn't hurt to continue consuming them. Sports drinks with added minerals may be better. Drinking fruit juices other than grapefruit in large amounts is not recommended because they contain a lot of sugars. In a recent study, children who drank an extra twelve ounces of juice a day tended to be shorter and heavier than their peers. Additionally, an excessive acid dose of the flouride in many juice preparations can destroy a youngster's tooth enamel. Colas should not be consumed in excess either. They contain carbonated water, phosphoric acid, and caffeine, and each of these alone, and certainly in combination, can produce osteoporosis (see page 290). I frequently recommend Fresca because it is non-phosphorated, has no carbohydrates, and does contain real grapefruit juice.

The only milk I recommend is mother's milk. Cow's milk is udderly unhealthy. Bovine casein, the milk protein, causes mischief in humans. It not only promotes osteoporosis, but in large amounts can also cause problems with the kidneys. The fat in milk, which is butter fat, elevates cholesterol and triglycerides. Furthermore, thirty percent of the adult population is lactose intolerant. They lack the enzyme, lactase, to break the milk sugar into its components, sucrose and fructose, to be easily absorbed. The resulting incomplete digestion causes gas, stomach cramps, bloating, and diarrhea. Yogurt, buttermilk, and hard cheese such as Swiss or cheddar have minimal lactose and can be consumed by those who are lactose intolerant. Oral lactase is available if we want to indulge in a bowl of ice cream or other milk products. Lastly, xanthine oxidase has recently been isolated from cow's milk and shown to cause arterial disease. In the process of homogenation all the fat globules are converted into small uniform ones which allow the them plus xanthine oxidase to be absorbed into our bloodstream even better to do damage.

## A Bridge Over Troubled Waters

Good, old-fashioned water, the universal solvent, should be the bulk of our liquid intake. In the twenty-first century, most water is no longer good, nor old-fashioned. Accounting for 70% of the cell's weight, it provides the environment that makes life possible. We are engineered around the special properties of water. Its polarity, ability to form hydrogen bonds, and surface tension regulate the free flow of water. In the human body, water resides in two molecular states — bound and the transiently clustered. Bound water is physically attached to other molecules and is more restricted from moving through our cell walls. As we age, the quantity of bound clustered water increases. Water coming from deep subterranean wells and in the polar ice caps has a greater proportion of micro clustered water molecules. Soon after exposed to air, it reverts to the normal larger clusters. Chlorine, an oxidizing agent, added to "purify" our drinking water, also does bodily injury. Several decades ago Dr. Joseph Fisher discovered that chlorinated water can promote cancer and arteriosclerosis. His studies were suppressed by the water industry and therefore are not commonly known. Just letting plain tap water sit in an open container for several hours will remove much of the dangerous chlorine. Running the tap for a minute to get rid of the first quart may decrease the contamination from the plumbing in the faucet which has more potential harmful effects per inch than plain pipes. One of the harmful byproducts of chlorinated tap water is trihalomethanes (THMs), known to be carcinogenic and abortive. A prominent environmental group reported that they found fecal coliform bacteria in 1,172 water systems nationwide, lead in 2,551 systems, and radioactive materials (such as radon) in 326 systems. Other studies show that at least forty-three percent of all water supplies violate federal standards, and as many as nine hundred die from waterborne diseases, such as cyrtospordium parvum. MTBE, a gasoline additive, may cause cancer and has been found in thousands of water supplies. I recommend drinking water that's been "decontaminated" by reverse osmosis or by distillation. A good silver impregnated charcoal filter on the faucet may be an alternative. In municipal waters, there is the Safe Drinking Water Hotline at 800-426-4791, or you can visit the website *www.epa.gov/safewater/dwinfo.htm.*

Another choice may be bottled water, which falls under the jurisdiction of the FDA adopted from the EPA standards for tap water. These waters, which may be from springs, wells, or just municipal city water, undergo purification by ozonization, reverse osmosis, a special "one-micron absolute filtration," and/or a special charcoal filter. These processes take out not only the impurities, but the disease-causing organisms. The tastes of these waters vary, not so much from the source, but material in which they are bottled. Those that come in PET plastic bottles generally taste better than the water that comes in HDPE. Some products contain natural minerals, such as the best natural spring water costing thirty cents for an eight-ounce glass with no off taste. Others have the minerals, particularly magnesium, added back, such as found in *Sam's's Choice* for six cents a glass.

Water is naturally found in a lattice cluster formation with dozens of molecules. The bigger the cluster, the more inefficient that water is in hydrating our individual cells. The most efficient and smallest cluster possible is that with a five molecular group known as a water pentamer. A product, Penta-Hydrate™, meets this qualification. The pentamer water causes a lower surface tension with the small cluster resulting in a wetter water with better transportation of these molecules through the pores of our cells, carrying both oxygen and nutrients more efficiently. This water operates as an antioxidant binding and neutralizing free radicals. According to the manufacturer, people experience increased stamina and feel better. This water is pricey. However, it is worked in with other less expensive water, so just one to two eight-ounce bottles a day are enough. Recommended that a half to full bottle upon rising and then some before meals, with daily vitamin and herbal supplements, as well as before, during, and after exercising. Additionally, Penta-Hydrate™ alleviates fatigue and improves the immune system. If interested, more information or the product can be obtained by calling 800-531-5088 or by visiting the website *www.hydrateforlife.com.*

## Coffee for Me

For the past thirty years I have reviewed study after study of the pros and cons of drinking coffee. Some research implicates caffeine as the culprit, and some points to coffee itself. Regarding caffeine, some folks experience cardiac arrhythmias (irregular and rapid heartbeats) from this chemical; others feel nervous and jittery during the day and are unable to sleep at night. In a 1998 study published in *Psychosomatic Medicine,* Dr. James Lane at Duke University noted that drinking four to five cups of regular coffee a day boosted the blood pressure of volunteers up five points compared to the days they drank just one cup. The pressure remained elevated for twelve hours. The author speculated that over the decades this slight increase of blood pressure could take its toll in premature cardiovascular disease. The most bad news comes from research showing that coffee elevates the level of homocysteine in the blood. This raises significantly the risk of coronary artery disease, stroke, and all cause deaths. Fortunately, paper coffee filters mitigate most of these harmful effects. In a study published in the *American Journal of Nutrition* in 2000 [71(2): 480-84] the unfiltered brew elevated the homocysteine level by twenty percent in a month, compared to when the same individuals drank filtered coffee eight weeks later. Paper filters remove the diterpenes in the coffee that both elevate homocysteine and increase cholesterol production. It made no difference if the coffee was decaffeinated or not. Thus, if one must drink coffee, I recommend moderate (one to three cups a day) consumption using a double paper filter.

Coffee does have some health benefits, too. The grounds remove eighty-five percent of the lead and copper from tap water! They may also capture other heavy metals such as mercury, cadium, and zinc. Coffee may prevent or decrease gallstones, Rheumatoid arthritis, and Parkinson's disease. Lastly, there is no definite evidence that coffee causes cancer.

## Tea for Two

In the *American Journal of Epidemiology* in 1999 H.D. Hesse explains that with or without caffeine, tea is a beneficial drink. Green tea, because of its phenolic content and many flavonoids, has been touted in China as being healthful for at least two millennia. Its phytochemicals disarm toxic free-radicals by chelating (grabbing) iron and copper, which slows down the generating of new diseases. It protects against cancer infections and aging according to a recent JAMA article. Another group of researchers at Purdue found that EGCg, a potent antioxidant in the tea, disables an enzyme that cancer cells need to divide and reproduce. In another article published in *The American Journal of Clinical Nutrition* (1999: 1040-1050), Dr. Dulloo at the University of Geneva in Switzerland made further claims that green tea helps shed fat pounds by increasing thermogenesis. Black tea, which comes from the same plant but is processed differently, may be just as good. To obtain the healthy benefits of the antioxidants in tea, brew it for only two or three minutes. Longer brewing makes a stronger tea, but does not increase its antioxidant activity. Tea, be it black or green, is protective against coronary artery disease. Tea can be served hot or cold. (See page 199.) Of course, there are also many herbal teas that have different properties, depending on the plant that is used, that are refreshing and even healthful.

## Alcohol

Alcohol may be consumed, but it is a double-edged sword. Too much of it impairs thinking and motor skills, decreasing our ability to operate machinery (including vehicles) safely. On the other hand, its beneficial effects include raising the good cholesterol (HDL), decreasing blood-clotting factors that can cause heart attacks, improving some individual social graces, as well as accentuating relaxation. Certainly, if a patient has a tendency to over-drink, a family history of alcoholism, or religious conflicts, he or she should avoid alcohol. Operation of heavy equipment or driving even after one drink more than offsets any benefit.

Alcohol is a plant product, and therefore, a carbohydrate full of calories (seven per gram). Thus, if a person drinks, he or she must decrease overall food intake to avoid getting fat. Consumed in excess, alcohol can raise the blood triglycerides, and place fat in the liver in some susceptible individuals.

Chronic excess leads to many health problems including elevated blood pressure and uric acid, and over a long period of time, tissue damage in the liver (cirrhosis), muscles, brain, and heart. Women, because of their metabolic differences, should generally drink half as much alcohol as men.

Wine, particularly the reds, would be my recommendation because they contain a variety of antioxidants and are more beneficial than other types of alcoholic products. No more than six ounces should be drunk in a ninety-minute period, and only while eating, since food slows down the absorption of alcohol. Antioxidants like resveratol, which is most concentrated in Pinot Noir, are produced by grapes to ward off infecting invaders to the fruit. In humans, resveratol has been shown to stimulate nerve cell connections and may be helpful in Alzheimer's Disease. Resveratol has been isolated and sold in capsules, and is also found in dark grape juice, although its concentration is half that of wine. Neither of these alcohol-free sources are as effective as red wine, however.

Wine has further health benefits as well. A major Harvard study conducted by Dr. Gary Curham showed that of 81,093 women ages forty to sixty-five, those who had a daily eight-ounce glass of wine reduced the risk of having kidney stones by fifty-nine percent. The same amount of tea, regular, or decaffeinated coffee would reduce the risk by only nine percent. Recently, beer has also been shown to prevent kidney stones, as well as osteoporosis. Scientists believe the hops in beer were the beneficial agent.

**Figure 3-XI.**

**Life's Weighty Problems**

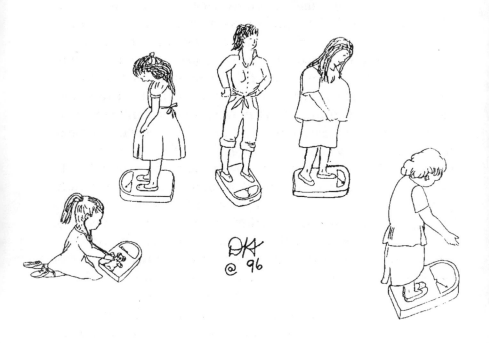

**To try is to fail. To do is to succeed.**

# FOUR

# Forever Young

## THE PROBLEM

YOU ARE GOING TO DIE! We as humans will not win that war. However, armed with prudent and healthy living, combined with the facts we now know to be effective and what we surmise to be helpful in the future, we will win many battles and postpone the final encounter. This will enable us to have the quality (live better) and quantity (live longer). In the year 2001, one out of three babies born will be a centurian.

As a physician, I have often wondered if we should consider aging a disease and treat it as such. Certainly both primary and secondary aging are under genetic control. There certainly are well described premature aging diseases such as Progeria (the body of a 20-year-old is functionally 80), and Alzheimer's disease (premature aging of the mind). On the other hand, the Methuselah gene was predicted in 1992. This is responsible for the cellular production of a powerful antioxidant, superoxide desmutase (S.O.D), in which one could stay physically young until they are 100. The genetic aspect of aging is being worked out in The Human Genome Project, which is determining the site of each of 3.2 billion genes. This is the code of all codes, *ours*. It should be finished by the time this book is published.

The human genome sequence will be the foundation of biology for decades and centuries to come. It is comparable to the periodic elemental table initiated over a century ago and was the basis for the discovery of almost a hundred new elements to include radioactive ones that lead to nuclear energy production. Already, researchers are extracting DNA (gene material) from persons blood, attaching fluorescent molecules and sprinkling it on a special glass chip. This chip has its surface sprinkled with 15,000 known genes. A laser reads the fluorescence, which indicates which of the known genes on the chip are in the mystery sample from patient. This gene expression will give us the power to re-engineer the human species and gradually improve the quality of life by attacking both secondary (degenerative) diseases and primary (just getting old) aging. The three plus billion genes are on 23 paired chromosomes (alleles) which are labeled as chromosome 1, chromosome 2, etc, and the two sex chromosomes identified as x and y. For premature aging CSA (Cockayne syndrome) on chromosome 5 and WRN (Werner Syndrome) on chromosome 8 have been located. For secondary aging IDDM 1 (diabetes of juvenile onset) on 6, IDDM 2 (adult onset diabetes) on 11, PS1-AD3 (Alzheimer's) on 14, MLH1 (colon cancer) on 3, plus 72 other diseases positions have been determined. Protgeonomics has emerged from genomics with the discovery that one gene can make at least ten different proteins.

Many potential diseases will hence be cured on a molecular level even before they arise. Pharmacogenetics, a recently recognized science will indicate just not how an individual will metabolize a drug (fast or slow), but whether a given drug will work for an individual patient. One also can prevent a gene from making a harmful protein such as the B-amyloid of Alzheimer's disease by bombarding (injecting) "antisense" molecules to foil the protein production. Therefore, aging is a definite but not an immutable process of living.

On a cellular level, at birth our cells are programmed to multiply only so many times before they individually die. This highly organized form of cell death is critical for both our health and our demise. When the process malfunctions, too little programmed cell death results in cancer or auto immune diseases, while too much causes acceleration of the degenerative diseases. This natural programmed cell death is called *apoptosis*. At the end of the process suicide is committed by the cell, chopping themselves into membrane-wrapped chunks. Cells compose tissues which accumlatively make up our organs. And of course, we are made up of organs (heart, kidney, lungs, etc.). Natural decline of our cells (tissues and organs) is aging and adding an insult to injury with degenerative disease processes could result in a catastrophic event for that organ system, causing death of the human being.

We do not doubt our beliefs, but we do believe our doubts. A recent survey by the Harvard School of Public Health shows that most of us have a pessimistic statistic about certain diseases. For example, women put their odds of developing breast cancer at 40 percent, whereas it is 10 percent. Men say that prostate cancer strikes down 30 percent, but the truth is only 10 percent get the disease. Being seriously injured in an auto accident, people felt was 50 percent when it is actually at 5 percent. Nearly everyone doubled their risk of getting stroke, heart attack, diabetes or HIV from the true statistic. Life expectancy certainly has increased in the last century, but most of this is not due to breakthroughs in treating disease by our high tech methods, but primarily due to better obstetrical techniques, improvement in prenatal mortality, and control of infectious diseases in childhood through immunization. It is true that we have pushed the envelope a little and postponed death by expensive procedures such as bypass surgery. Although as mentioned above we are breaking our genetic way, but most of the prolongation of life in the near future will be through preventive methods such as intervening early in our genetic determinates, advertising against smoking, eating excessively, being sedentary, and by keeping a "clean" house. The latter includes drinking clean water (see page 99), carbon filters in faucets and showerheads, keeping the kitchen fan on while running hot water or emptying the dish washer, and waiting a few hours after the last dish washer cycle completes before opening. Also, wash clothes in cold water, in that hot water releases more chlorine into the air. Do heavy loads of wash, which keeps the sloshing and agitation to a minimum that reduces the transfer of chemicals to the air. If possible, keep laundry facilities in the part of the house away from people. Avoid mothballs, toilet and personal deodorants. Store household chemicals (cleaners, pesticides, etc) outside the house structure, not in an attached garage or not as most, under the kitchen sink. Avoiding exposure to electromagnetic waves from portable phones, many electric devices and in particular microwave ovens will also extend life. These insults to the human body are cumulative. Therefore, the longer and the more agents the more the damage. Air dry-cleaned clothes well before wearing them. In the past, the medical field's best intervention was to recognize and control hypertension, but we are now far ahead of this

As was mentioned above, it is not just living longer, but living better. My patients often say to me that they don't want to live and be old with all the hardships it entails. But on the other hand, who wants to be old when one is still relatively young? I know people in their 50's who feel old and sick, and others in their 80's who are healthy and spry. It is not how old you are chronologically (your age), but how old you are physically (your internal functions and external appearance) that counts.

We do have to get older, but we do not have to age as we get older. But genetically and even biblically speaking (Genesis 6:3), we should live to be 120. To examine how to live longer, we need to look into why certain individuals such as Jean Calmet of France died at age 122 in 1997. This then is studying the oldest of the old such as the government-funded study currently being done in Baltimore. Medicine explains it nicely, degenerative diseases, super imposed or primary aging. A machine, even a human one, will not last forever. We know that infection, trauma, heart disease and cancer do cause our demise, but even if there are none of these, primary aging will kill us. It is a fact of life that we will all die hence the old adage, "The two basic truths in life are, we will pay taxes and we will die," despite the new tax law that we will not have to pay *as* much tax when we die. So, we will all die sometime. Hopefully, that time will be when we are close to our six score years.

A long life is not necessarily synonymous with a healthy one, but I want to discuss a long, healthy life as was the design of our Creator; then, suddenly, Peace, Oblivion, Heaven, or whatever your belief system is. Whether it is the "Big Bang Theory" and evolution, or that God made the earth and all within it, including us, is a moot point. That we are here from chance, luck, or as I feel, through God, makes little difference. But, the fact is that we *are* here and should and can live life to its fullest and at its best. Many of us feel that we don't mind death, but do mind dying!, or, as the late George Burns said, "I don't want to be there when it happens." Therefore, it is not with prolonging death, but prolonging life and all the goodness it entails; and then that sudden and perhaps beautiful transition to the hereafter, or what some personally feel will be our "life after death.

## THE IMPACT OF DISEASE

Disease certainly will change the ideal life curve (Fig. 4-I) to what we typically see today or even being pessimistically optimistic within the next decade. Some diseases are promptly announced at the beginning of the process such as an overwhelming infection like pneumonia. But others are very subtle like atherosclerosis, and it is years or even decades before they become noisy and, hence, recognized. Defeating the disease process as it first gets started, or better yet, before it is introduced into our tissue such as in embryo or at birth should be medicine's goal. This could be accomplished more and more by family history or genetic testing of cord blood at birth. Then, hopefully, we can take measures to reverse (gene therapy), to prevent or greatly retard the course of disease. In describing life, we need to consider both morbidity and vitality. Morbidity and vitality are inversely related. Therefore 100 percent vitality has no morbidity and conversely. Certainly, there is no vitality in death (mortality), which is 100 percent morbid. The graph (see Fig. 4-II) may help to detail this better. An earlier identification and a therapeutic intervention (see Fig. 4-III) will decrease morbidity and prevent mortality.

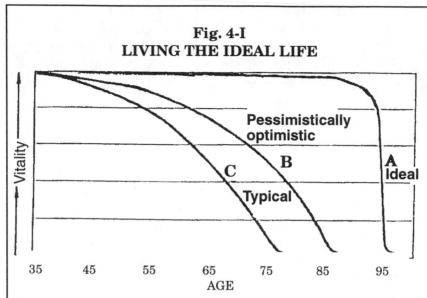

**The Ideal Life Curve**

A.  The "ideal" life curve illustrates the notion that healthy hab-
    its can sustain vitality and good health over a long life, with
    a brief and precipitous decline near the very end.

B.  A somewhat less optimistic view holds that while it may be
    possible to delay the decline, it generally can't be put off that
    far or compressed that much.

C.  The typical course in the year 2001.

It is far better if a disease is detected, stop it, live a full
life (see Fig. 4-III) and wake up dead at age 110. On the
other side of the coin, this is not what we have today. A degenerative disease process such as atherosclerosis (see Fig.
4-II) may have its onset at age 20 and slowly progress —
because of genetic or environmental reasons such as smoking or unhealthy diet — to age 50. With the change of

## Fig. 4-II
## A REAL LIFE CURVE

A — Disease Onset        A-C — Silient Disease
C — Crisis — First (Symptoms)    C-I — Noisy Disease
E — Crisis — Second
I _ Death

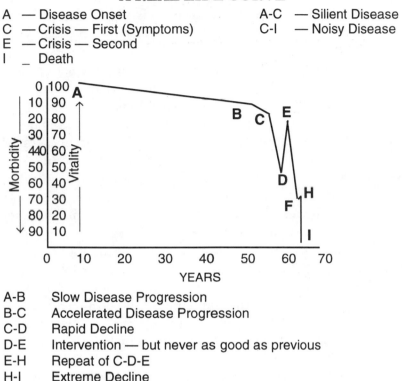

A-B    Slow Disease Progression
B-C    Accelerated Disease Progression
C-D    Rapid Decline
D-E    Intervention — but never as good as previous
E-H    Repeat of C-D-E
H-I    Extreme Decline

## Fig. 4-III
## A SQUARE LIFE CURVE

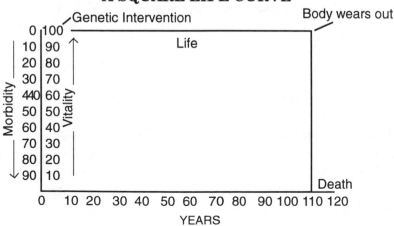

lifestyle, with being more sedentary, having more stress (financial, marital, having a teenager, etc.), the atherosclerosis accelerates. At age 58, the disease is diagnosed, perhaps by going to the doctor because of chest pain and high cholesterol. The atherosclerosis process still progresses, but medical intervention helps some and there is some improvement. Then comes "the big one," a heart attack at age 60, which markedly alters one's health. The person survives, but has congestive heart failure. Subsequent to his injured heart muscle, he is hospitalized, but makes it. However, he is never as well as he was before. The survival is only temporary, and within six months of a miserable existence in a nursing home, he dies! Again, returning to Fig. 4-III, with an earlier diagnosis, we can nip the disease in the bud and compact the mortality to a very short time before death.

It is that persons last small fraction of his life that cost not only an inordinate amount of health care dollars, but for that poor individual an unbearable amount of misery. The patient, as well as the immediate family indeed suffers. These misfortunes then do not prolong life, but prolong the unhappy ending to what otherwise might be a full and rewarding life.

Presently, as we get older, we have more and more illnesses, which leave us more and more feeble, and hence we have a lingering death. We have all heard the expression that a patient looks like "death warmed over." The patient looks old, feels old and, indeed, is chronologically old. The gradual descent into old age, older age, and then death is what is happening to most of us today. The ideal would be to be healthy until the last day or two of our existence and then die, or better yet, go to sleep one night and "wake up dead." Disability and functional impairment will be compressed to a very brief time after an extremely lengthy period of health and vigor. In the *New England Journal of Medicine*, April 9, 1998, Dr. Anthony Vita examined data from the 1941 alumni of the University of Pennsylvania born between 1913 and 1925. The relationship to modifiable factors of smoking, body mass index and exercise pattern indicated that better health habits not only increase survival, but more importantly, postpone and compress disability to a shorter time at life's end. The time to be concerned about when and how we die is now while there is still time to do something about it.

## THE BIOLOGY OF AGING

Aging can be divided in to a primary and secondary condition. Primary aging at the cellular level can be defined as a progressive deterioration of structure and function that occurs over time. Secondary aging is the superimposition of degenerative processes that progress with time. These include such entities as atherosclerosis, osteoarthritis, Alzheimer's diseases, and all the handicaps that occur with them. Healthy or successful aging is the delaying of the cellular deterioration and the prevention of degradation. Shortly we will discuss the theories of aging, but restricting food intake, exercise and hormone replacement have definitely been proven in the medical literature to retard primary aging humans. In a symposium published in the Mayo Clinic Proceedings in mid-2000 just testosterone replacement in the elderly, will retard both primary and secondary aging.

We all live to die, but some of us are dying to live. The last of life is far better if one continues enthusiasm, which will help ensure longevity. It is contentment, complacency and satisfaction not the excitement and the exhilaration that is important for lengthening our pleasurable life span. People do age at different rates and even within a given individual a given organ system exhibits varying speeds of decline. Aging occurs throughout our body: the heart rate and force of contraction decrease, blood vessel diameter decreases, muscles lose mass, bones develop osteoporosis, lung capacity diminishes, skin loses collagen, hormonal production changes dramatically, and there are significant alterations in sensory functions. Some researchers refer to the pause of an organ system, such as the menopause, as a sudden decline in the ovaries of a woman as a reflection of aging. The earlier the identification of the multiple pauses that comprise primary aging, the earlier and simpler the intervention will be and the more successful the outcomes. In the following discussion I will detail the skin and the eyes more because of limitation of space.

## AGING OF OUR BODY PARTS

**Brain**: Some scientists believe aging begins in the brain with "electropause," a change in the P300, the positive brain wave, at 300ms. The loss of amplitude and/or voltage results in delays of neurotransmission in the cortex, with implications for every body organ and system. Over time, the brain loses some neurons and others become damaged. The brain adapts to these changes, however, by increasing the number of synapses and by regenerating dendrites and axons. However, there is a toll with decrease memory and reaction time as the brain electrically and structurally ages. Neurobiofeedback using a computer program with an electroencephalogram is definitely useful in retarding brain aging.

**Eye**: Essential for good sight is early detection of glaucoma, prevention and treatment of macular degeneration, cataract interception and control of blood sugar in diabetes. Both macular degeneration and cataracts may be prevented by antioxidants. The former demands early and intensive treatment, where as the latter can continue until vision reaches a critical point, then surgery. Since we are as young as we look and feel, having good eyesight particularly without glasses is valuable in staying younger, longer. First we will discuss refractive problems which is the main reason we need glasses particularly before the age of 60. Then we will address glaucoma, cateract, diabetic eye disease, and macular degeneration. Your grandmother may be correct that highly colored vegetables are good for your eyesight, but reading in low light will not adversely affect vision. However, vision problems can make it difficult to read in low light.

**Refractive Correcting Procedure** — All refractive corneal surgery reshapes the cornea to redirect light rays so that they focus on the retina. In myopia, (near sightedness) rays converge in front of the retina; surgical flattening of the cornea focuses the rays farther back. In hyperopia, (far sightedness) light rays strike the retina before they can focus; steepening the cornea makes the rays converge closer to the retina. In astigmatism, the cornea is not spherical because one meridian is steeper or flatter than the others; flattening a steep meridian or steepening a flat meridian tends to bring the light rays in focus nearer to the retina. The poor focusing of an image does cause blurring of our vision as do other eye diseases. The following will give name and particular corrective procedure. Also visit the popular website, *www.fda.gov/cdrh/lasik.*

LASIK — In laser in-situ keratomileusis, the surgeon uses a microkeratome to make a thin flap in the cornea. An excimer laser programmed to correct the patient's myopia, hyperopia and/or astigmatism is used to etch away a predetermined pattern of corneal tissue from the tissue beneath the flap, which is then repositioned without suturing. Following the procedure, most patients have little discomfort and recover vision within 48 hours. From 5% to 30% require a second lifting of the flap and reshaping of the cornea, usually three to six months after the first procedure. Lasik does not correct loss of accommodation with aging, so most folks will still need reading glasses. Over-corrections and under-corrections occur, but they can often be corrected with retreatment. Irregular astigmatism that decreases vision can also occur. Glare and halos around lights at night are frequent after Lasik. They tend to disappear after a few months, but some patients may continue to have vision problems at night or in dim lighting.

PRK — Photorefractive keratectomy is similar to Lasik in using a laser to reshape the stromal surface of the cornea, but does so without a corneal incision or use of a flap. The laser itself ablates the corneal epithelium, and re-epithelialization is required to cover the defect after surgery. Overall results are similar to those with Lasik. PRK can cause considerable postoperative discomfort because of the epithelial defect. Other relative disadvantages are prolonged recovery of vision, the difficulty of performing subsequent corrective procedures, and central haziness caused by sub-epithelial healing. As with Lasik, glare and halos around lights can be a problem. Unlike Lasik, which is usually done to both eyes in a single procedure, PRK is usually done separately on the two eyes, with an interval of four to six weeks.

RK — In radial keratomy, deep radial incisions created with a diamond scapel weaken the peripheral part of the cornea, causing the peripheral cornea to bulge outward and the central cornea to become flatter. RK is rarely performed today.

INTRACORNEAL RINGS — The FDA last year approved the implantation of polymethyl-methacrylate (PMMA) ring segments (*Intacs* – Keravision) into the peripheral cornea to flatten the anterior curvature of the central cornea and correct low degrees of the myopia (up to 3 Diopters). PMMA is the same material used for the lens implants in cataract surgery. Correction is achieved by reshaping the outer edge of the cornea. About two thirds of patients have achieved 20/20 vision or better with this procedure. An advantage of the intracorneal rings is that they can be removed, usually restoring the eye to its preoperative refractive error, or replaced with a different-size ring, making this potentially an adjustable procedure. New configurations of the rings are under development for treating astigmatism and possibly hyperopia. Common complications include mild postoperative pain and occasional glare at night.

PHAKIC INTRAOCULAR LENSES — Recent improvements in intraocular lens lens technology now permit implantation of plastic intraocular lenses without removing the natural crystalline lens. These lenses are under investigation for correction of high myopia and hyperopia and may be the procedure of the future as the technology improves.

**Glaucoma**: The symptoms of glaucoma are visual loss and blurred vision. Glaucoma, a partial loss of ones view, caused by increased pressure in the eye fluid that damages the optic nerve. It affects one million Americans 65 and older and is the leading cause of blindness among African Americans. Eight out of 10 glaucoma cases are the open angle type and account for 10% of cases of legal blindness in the U.S. Risk factors include family history, increased age, extreme near-sightedness, hypertension, diabetes, and long-term corticosteroid therapy. The disease develops more frequently and earlier among African Americans, and may be detected as early as age 40. Patients often remain asymptomatic until the disease ahs progressed significantly. The American Academy of Ophalmology recommends that people older than 45 undergo comprehensive eye examinations every two years, and every year if they have risk factors for glaucoma. Closed angle glaucoma develops in 20% of cases and is more symptomatic and dangerous. Several types of medications and/or surgery may reduce intraocular pressure.

**Cataract**: The symptoms are blurred vision, glare, and double vision. Opacitites in the lens of the eye, or cataracts, affect fewer than 5% of persons under 65, but almost half of Americans 75 and older. *The Archives of Opthalmology* (2000; 118 1556-63) reported people taking Vitamins C and E for greater than ten years had a 60% reduced risk of cataracts. The most common cause of blindness worldwide, cataracts are a less important cause of vision impairment in the United States because of the availability and efficacy of outpatient cataract surgery. More than 1.5 million such procedures are performed each year, and 90% of treated patients enjoy a significant visual improvement, with a 1% complication rate. These are several types of procedures. Choose the ophthalmologist who has done hundreds of them and has a good reputation.

**Diabetic (Retinopathy) Eye Disease**: The symptoms are blurred vision, floaters, visual field loss, and poor right vision. Anyone with diabetes or prediabetes, such as the elevated blood sugar of syndrome X may develop diabetic eye disease. Diabetic retinopathy affects many middle-aged and older Americas, who are at risk of Type 2 diabetes. Diabetic retinopathy may escape detection for some time. Ten to twenty percent of people diagnosed with Type 2 diabetes concurrently have retinopathy. Patients who complain of blurry vision or distorted central vision may have "background" or nonproliferative diabetic retinopathy which is caused by hemorrhages or a fluid collection. Proliferative diabetic retinopathy involves the growth of new, abnormal blood vessels in the retina that leak, impair vision, and may cause retinal detachment. Various surgical approaches and laser treatment are effective in both forms of diabetic retinopathy. In people with diabetes, good blood sugar control is believed to prevent or delay the onset of diabetic retinopathy and slow its progression once it has occurred.

**Macular degeneration**: Macular degeneration affects more than 15 million people in the U.S. The macula is a small area in the retina, which is needed for central vision. This is the focus used to view fine work, such as reading and sewing. Higher risk is noted in smokers, over exposure to sunlight, women and persons with lighter colored (blue, green and hazel) eyes. Cataracts of varying degree frequently accompany macular degeneration. There are two types; the wet, which occurs in 10 percent of the people with macular degeneration, and the dry which, is noted in the remaining 90%. The wet is much more aggressive and gets its name from the bleeding capillaries within the macula. The dry type usually progresses over years or decades, is caused by deterioration of the macular cells. These are pigmented and it seems that blue light causes their dysfunction, and later destruction.

Antioxidants, zeaxanthin, lutein (page 233, Omega 3 fish oils (page 74, and zinc (page182) retard and/or prevent dry macular degeneration. For the wet variety, laser has been used to stop the capillary bleeding, but also destroys some of the good capillaries and other cells. An old technique has been refined for the treatment of the wet disease. The drug is called Verteporfin (Visudyne®). It is given intravenously and the ophthalmologist targets the vessel with a low power laser that "turns on" the drug which causes micro blood clots in the small vessels and hence, seals them off. This treatment is extremely effective in 30 percent of those with wet

## Figure 4-IV

**DO YOU HAVE MACULAR DEGENERATION?**

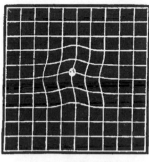 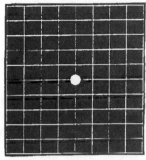

Abnormal                  Normal

**Testing your vision with the Amsler grid:**
You can check your vision daily by using an Amsler grid like the one pictured above on the right. You may find changes in your vision that you wouldn't notice otherwise. Xeroxing or cutting the grid and putting it on the front of your refrigerator is a good way to remember to look at it each day, or just open to this page. There is both a wet (more rapid and severe) and a dry (more common) type.

**To use the grid:**
1. Wear your reading glasses and hold this grid at 12-15 inches in good light.
2. Cover one eye.
3. Look directly at the center dot with the uncovered eye.
3. While looking directly at the center dot, note whether all lines of the grid are straight or if any areas are distorted, blurred or dark as the one on the left.
5. Repeat this procedure with the other eye.
6. If any area of the grid looks wavy, blurred or dark, such as on the left, contact your ophthalmologist immediately.

macular degeneration. Recently, intravenous injections of EDTA (Chelation) have been shown to be effective in both dry and wet macular degeneration, as well as for cataracts. See Figure IV to determine if you have macular degeneration. Blurred vision, image distortion, and holes in the visual field are symptoms of macular degeneration. Using the grid frequently will allow you to determine if you have this disease and then seek immediate ophthalmologic care.

**Heart**: The heart grows slightly larger with age. Maximal oxygen consumption during exercise declines in men by about 10 percent and in women by about 7.5 percent with each decade of adult life. Cardiac output stays nearly the same, however, because the heart actually pumps more efficiently.

**Lungs**: Maximum breathing capacity may decline by about 40 percent between the ages of 20 and 80 years.

**Blood vessels**: Arterial walls thicken and systolic blood pressure increases 20-25 percent between ages 20 and 75 years. This hardening and rusting of the pipes is referred to as a "vasculopause."

**Pancreas**: A decline in this organ might be called an "Insulopause." Glucose metabolism declines progressively, as measured by glucose tolerance tests.

**Kidneys**: These organs gradually become less efficient at extracting wastes from the blood. The associated organs are also effective. Bladder capacity declines. Urinary incontinence, which may occur after tissues atrophy, can often be managed through exercise hormone and behavioral techniques. The prostate enlarges, but can be treated with Proscar™ , or Saw Palmetto (see page 207). Some antiaging specialists refer to this as the "Uropause."

**Body fat**: The body does not lose fat with age but redistributes it from just under the skin to deeper parts of the body. Women are more likely to store it in the hips and thighs, while men store it in the abdominal area.

**Muscles**: Without exercise, estimated muscle mass declines 22 percent for women and 23 percent for men between the ages of 30 and 70. Hand grip strength decreases 45 percent by age 75. Exercise, especially resistance training, can help prevent much of this loss.

**Ears**: Ability to hear high-frequency tones begins to decrease as early as age 20. Low-frequency hearing ability declines in the 60's. Between the ages of 30 and 80, men lose hearing more than twice as quickly as women. Rates of hearing loss are strongly influenced by intensity and duration of noise exposure.

**Personality**: After about age 30, personality tends to be stable. Sudden changes in personality frequently suggest the onset of a secondary disease process.

**Teeth**: Loss of the white protective enamel and discoloration of teeth occurs. Not only do the dental structures recede, but the gums surrounding them do as well, and the person is literally "long in tooth." The teeth are more brittle and, since the roots are stronger than the tooth, breakage and losing teeth are the consequence.

**Bone**: As we get older, our bones become more brittle because of the loss of minerals and protein (see page 289).

**Smell/Taste**: The nerves that supply the nose with oral factory sense decrease starting around 30, and 50 percent of the sense of smell is gone by age 80. Since taste is appreciated on the tongue (salt, sweet, sour, bitter), along with the smell, it is lost as well.

**Skin**: To sustain a youthful appearance, patients must address the systemic effects of age on the body. Long-term lifestyle factors as well as anti-aging nutrients and hormones will provide the most benefit to preserve or restore youthful skin and hair. Hair will be discussed later in this chapter. Apart from the relentless ticking of the biological clock, much skin aging results from exposure to ultraviolet (UV) radiation from the sun, both UVA and UVB. The tanning beds are also very harmful to the skin, producing lots of bad UVA radiation. To maintain youthful skin, it is best to avoid direct sunlight whenever possible, and wear protection when exposed. A good sunscreen is probably the most important long-term topical anti-aging preparation. Taking PABA internally also offers some UV protection.

UV and free oxygen radicals combine to stimulate the synthesis of collagenase, an enzyme that degrades collagen, without stimulating synthesis of an anti-collagenase. The latter prevents collagen degradation. Eventually, this imbalance leads to the breakdown of collagen fibers in the skin's extracellular matrix, resulting in skin that sags. Also, sun destroys some of the all-important immunity of our skin.

Some studies have established that topically applied antioxidants can fight free radical damage in skin cells. As one example, topical applications of Vitamin E and asorbyl palmitate, the oil-soluble form of Vitamin C, are proven effective in controlled studies. A few other topicals such as Kinerase, have shown, in clinical studies, to combat photo-aging from sun. Other topical preparations can stimulate collagen formation. Dipalmityl hydroxy proline, also known as ASC III, promotes production of Collagen 3, the form of collagen most responsible for healing wounds. Collagen 3 constitutes most of a baby's skin but drops dramatically with advancing age. Brushing also tends to keep the skin younger. Also stimulating collagen production is epidermal growth factor (EGF), a protein produced by injured skin that enables it to heal itself by causing rapid generation of new cells. Creams containing EGF facilitate wound repair and support skin cell renewal. However, speaking anonymously, several estheticians and chemists interviewed at the recent Long Beach Beauty Show expressed concern that stimulating cell growth has potential to stimulate undesirable growth, such as malignant cells sold.

Jan Marini of *Jan Marini Research*, a company started by her, and who is a phenomenal esthetician that I have had the pleasure to meet, has shown that transformational growth factor stimulates collagen and elastin production. This enables wounds to heal and helps reverse visible signs of aging. Some preparations, such as extracts of sunflower seeds, claim to fight nonenzymic glycation. This cross linking of collagen that destroys skin elasticity and creates a tough, wrinkled texture often begins with the chemical attachment of glucose to skin collagen. There are also many health-based treatments that providers can offer to improve aging skin, including masks, wraps, detoxifiers and electrical stimulators that improve both muscle and skin tone. Visibly sagging and wrinkled skin signals a much greater health hazard, undesirable cross linking of tissues in organs, the underlying tissues and cells. Since we are as young as we look, keeping our skin young will keep us young. The use of Renova™ retards and in some cases reversed age spots and wrinkles. The Langerhan cell living in our skin is a literal army tank. It waits patiently and when a noxious infiltrating chemical, an invading organism such as bacteria or a single abnormal cancer cell is accidentally produced. "Sargent Langerhan" takes them out. UV light irreversibly harms this important immunity cellular form of skin protection. Hence, discoloration of the skin, infection and cancers do occur more.

Rejuvination of the skin can be accomplished by the fruit acid, glycolic acid. In high concentrations it is applied by a physician or prescribed for home use, but in lesser concentration put on by an esthetician and is available in a very diluted amount in cosmetics. Phenol had been used in the past, but has been replaced by glycolic acid and laser surgery and botulism, toxin (Botox) injections. These are done by a plastic surgeon, although many other physicians, some of whom are not qualified are doing the procedure. Acupuncture recently has come on to the American nonwrinkling scene and is less expensive and as effective as Botox. The ultimate is plastic surgery, which if done needs to be repeated every five to ten years.

**Hair:**To have a full head of hair will decrease the age of a male by as much as a decade. Hair loss is inevitable for both male and females as we get older. However, it's much more common and severe in men. Every decade after the age of 30, there is another 10% of the male population that loses significant hair. That is 30% of men over 40, 60% of men over 60, and 80% of men over 80. More important, the younger the individual when the hair is lost, the more significant it personally is. There is a genetic predisposition inherited from *both* parents indicating the hair loss gene is on at least two chromosomes. In addition to the genetics, hormones, too much sunlight, and recently discovered bacterial infection influence the incidence and rapidity of hair loss. The hormone is the androgen, testosterone, or more importantly its metabolite, dihydrotestosterone. Hence, it is referred to as *androgenetic alopecia*. The latter word is Greek for male hereditary hair loss.

The specifics of hair growth and loss is that hair normally grows in two to six year cycles. There is *anagen, the* growing phase that lasts two to five years; *catagen,* the regression phase lasting two to three weeks; and *telogen, the* resting phase that lasts three to four months. So at any one time, hair is always coming out. In male pattern baldness, the cycles do change with anagen reduced to only six to eight weeks and telogen lasting for years. Over the years, the hair becomes progressively thinner, finer, shorter and less pigmented. On the scalp initially this appears as thinning and later, balding. This is noticed by the patient with more hair on the pillow in the morning, hair in the shower drain, and if the individual or the doctor were to look at the hair, he would see a small club at the end of the hair indicating that this is the resting or telogen phase.

There are three letter presentations of balding; one, an "O" on the vertex, the top of the crown; another, which is more of the typical pattern where there is an "M" with the mid part of the M pointing to the nose. This is called bitemporal recession. Lastly, the anterior pattern where a "C"-shape referred to as anterior mid-scalp hair loss. As the hair loss continues, the front and back meet and there is just an edge of hair above the ears and around the back of the head.

In the twenty-first century, there are options to treat baldness, to include an aggressive surgical treatment with hair transplants, scalp reduction and rotation flaps. These are very effective, fairly expensive and for the most part, not paid by third party payers. Hairpieces, hair weaves, hair enhancers (shampoos, sprays, mousses), camouflaging (Derm Blend, which colors both the hair and the scalp) and approved medical therapies. The latter includes Propecia™ (finesteride), which is taken orally and Rogaine™

(Minoxidil), which is used topically on the scalp. Rogaine™ comes in both the 2% and 5% solution, is used twice a day, needs no prescription and is 50% effective in users. It has a 5% incidence of a rash after several weeks precluding its use. Propecia™ is by prescription only and has in its side effects, a decrease of libido. But, this has an incidence of less than 1%. Although we don't know exactly how Rogaine™ works, we do know how Propecia™ works. It inhibits the enzyme that converts the testosterone to the active form, dihydrotestosterone. The latter is a key factor in causing hair loss to genetically predisposed men, enlarging the prostate and perhaps producing prostate cancer. Both of these drugs take up to four months to see the benefits. These are lost two months after stopping the drugs. Rogaine™ costs about $70 for three months and Propecia™ costs about $125. These usually are not reimbursed by third party payers. To be more cost effective with Propecia™, which comes in a 1 mg size, one could purchase the 5mg Proscar™ (finesteride) by prescription, the *exact* same drug used to treat benign prostatic hypertrophy and take a fifth quarter of the drug daily. This will cut the price by 40 %. More than that, third party payers will pay for Proscar if the patient is so insured. Taking the 5 mg size will treat both prostate and hair loss. In that it is strongly suspected that bacteia similar to that found in acne could cause baldness, minocycline 100 mg twice a week or the less expensive doxycycline 100 mg a day may be helpful in addition to the above. Expert tattooing of bald spots on the scalp can camouflage some hair loss. Tattooing of eyebrows in both men and women who have premature grey or loss is also effective. Copper ingestion can in some cases return gray hair to its original color.

## THEORIES OF AGING

The Baltimore Longitudinal Study of Aging (BLSA) defines primary aging as the changes and processes that affect all people with time and can not be attributed to the diseases that accompany it. These illnesses as mentioned earlier are referred to as degenerative ones such as atherosclerosis. There is more theory than fact on the causes of aging. There are at least 20 theories, most of which have or will fall by the wayside. Those that have not, will be discussed in greater detail. In this chapter I'll give you my best thoughts on life extension. Those theories that are still regarded as plausible by researchers are detailed below.

In 1882, a German biologist, Dr. August Weisman, presented the *"Wear and Tear"* theory. In it our body and its components were damaged by use and abuse over time, just like a machine. Toxins in our environment, less than "healthy food," cosmic radiation, as well as physical and emotional stress shortened our life span. When we were young, our body could maintain and repair the damage we heaped upon it, and we were able to compensate for this. But as time moved on, we were unable to bring our very tissue, of which we were made, back to normal as when it was younger. Our immune system functioned less with time and we were prone to get overwhelming infections or cancer, for example.

Several researchers, 20 years ago, came out with the *"Waste Accumulation Theory"* in which, during the course of our normal metabolism, toxic products were produced which would build up. These substances were inherently damaging to our cells. Lipofuscin is such a chemical. It accumulates in cells as microscopic granules, and as they increase in size and number, make the cell function less than normal and, eventually, these cells die. We know this to be true in such diseases as Alzheimer's disease, any diseases of the heart and certain kidney diseases. There is a build-up of toxic material. So, if these chemicals were not produced, our aging and death would be retarded.

*"The Prenatal Conditioning Theory"* may be too late for us, but not for some of the younger generation. Dr. Peter Nathanelsz states that what happens in uterus can profoundly effect how one will be in life: yes, fetal programming can affect both the quality and the quantity of one's life. This Cornell University professor in a recent book, *"Live in the Womb,"* elaborates on the effect of pregnancy on the genetic code that was given at the dawn of conception. *"The*

*Telomerase Theory of Aging"* held a real promise for life extension. Telomerase is now being dubbed the immortality enzyme. This is the telomere-shortening hypothesis of senescence. A telomere is a piece of genetic material attached to the end of each chromosome, and looks like a shoelace with its end. The cell's senescence is characterized by shortening ever so slightly of the telomere with each cell division until it disappears. Then the cell can no longer divide and at the end of its finite life, it dies. In the Journal of Science (Jan. 16, 1998), studies on human cells show that a decreasing level of this enzyme leads to a gradual demise of chromosomes that ultimately stop cell division. At least in a test tube, we now can create immortal human cells by inhibiting the telomeres from shortening, by controlling the enzyme Telomerase

Planned obsolescence in the *"Genetic Control Theory"* indicated that our genes have encoded a predetermined tendency on how quickly or slowly we age. As the old adage goes: one way to live to be 100 years old is to pick parents who died when they were both 110 years old!! *"The Limited Number of Cell Division Theory"* was first promulgated by a French Nobel prize winner (1912), Dr. Alexis Carel, and improved upon by Dr. Leonard Hayflick and still later Dr. Paul Niehaus. The latest variation on this theory is that injection of extract of live fetal tissue will add to the number of cell divisions so they will divide and divide as long as this extract is given. *"The Thymic Stimulating Theory"* is advanced by Dr. Alan Goldstein, chairman of Biochemistry at George Washington University, who states that life depends on the thymus gland. Weighing 250 grams at birth, it gradually shrinks during life so that it weighs only 1/100 or 2.5 grams at age 60. The thymic hormones not only play a big role in how our immune system functions, but it also regulates our neurotransmitters (messengers of our nervous system) throughout our life. When our thymus gland shrinks too fast, we age prematurely. Live cell thymus, at least in experiments with animals, allows for increasing longevity.

*"The Mitochondrial Theory"* was first brought to light 40 years ago and languished until recently. In a study in *Sci-*

*ence,* October 22, 1999, investigators from the United States and Italy, using an extremely sensitive new technique, found specific malfunctioning of these microorgans (organelles) of our cells. It is these mitochondria that are the generators of energy in cells. As the mitochondria age from oxidative processes, the energy is reduced and stops. This results in weakened and subsequently death of our tissues. This study, which extended over a twenty-year period in some individuals, confirmed by DNA analysis what the electron microscope suspected decades earlier. *"The Death Hormone Theory"* or DECO (decreasing consumption of oxygen) states Dr. Donner Dencla, an endocrinologist, formerly at Harvard, regulates when we will die. This hormone is released by the pituitary gland as we get older and "poisons" our cells so we no longer use oxygen efficiently, and accelerates the aging process. Perhaps this hormone can be overcome by breathing more oxygen. This will, be discussed later (see page 133).

The theory that has the best press is *"The Free Radical Theory."* Although first proposed by Dunham Harman, M.D. in 1959 at the University of Nebraska, the free radical concept was not widely accepted until the mid-90's. Free radicals are very unstable organic compounds that seek out the very chemicals of which our body is structurally made, as well as other internal pathways of life. Examples of this include the fats which are then more rapidly incorporated into the plaque lining of our blood vessel walls, and which causes the DNA, the genetic make-up of our bodies, to be altered and damaged. These free radicals are generated in the normal process of oxygenation and respiration, of which the reaction continues slightly longer than it should. Our biochemical make-up is such that natural antioxidants neutralize these extra products of combustion like water putting out a fire that gets out of hand. When there is an excessive amount of oxidation, our natural processes are overwhelmed and the extra free radicals do damage to our tissues and the other natural substances in our body. To add insult to injury, not only do we produce free radicals naturally from doing our regular business of living and energizing our body (eating, digesting, metabolizing), but through the consumption and absorption of toxins in our water and in the air we breathe (smog, carbon dioxide, pesticides and cigarette smoke). Another recent development for the human race is in the depletion of the ozone layer that allows more cosmic radiation to do us more bodily harm than in the past.

As we age, the body sustains accumulative damage from oxidation. Our ability to neutralize the free radicals by the defending antioxidant buffers greatly diminishes. We have a natural, built-in method of antioxidizing products which are composed of enzymes (gluthiothione, catalase, SOD), vitamins (C, E, polyphenols, carotenoids, flavinoids) and trace minerals (selenium, zinc). The antioxidants quench the free radical fire produced in our body's furnaces as well as from external sources (cosmic radiation and toxins). The antioxidants scavenge the free radical particles and effectively neutralize them.

*"The Neuroendocrine Theory"* was initially developed by Vladimir Dilman Ph.D. and later adopted by thousands of physicians, including myself. This simply states that our endocrine glands function less as they get older. When their output ceases, so do we. These hormones are more or less regulated by the hypothalamus which directly stimulates the numerous hormones in what in the past was called the master gland — the pituitary. The hypothalamus, our internal clock, can be influenced by our external environment and hence, in a sense, can run faster or slower. Therefore, our sex hormones and growth hormones, among others, are all at the mercy of the hypothalamus. Perhaps the best studied theory is *"The Calorie Restriction Theory."* After decades of normal experiments, Dr. Roy Walford, a respected gerontologist at UCLA, documented that a high nutrient calorie diet, one where the subject borders on malnutrition, greatly prolongs life. This has also been shown in various other species such as water flies, spiders, guppies, rodents and chiggers. Both the Harvard Alumni Study by Dr. H. Lee as well as the Nurses Health Study by Dr. J. Manson, found that all cause mortality to be reduced by 20 percent in the lower

weight subjects compared to the national average. According to Dr. Richard Weinbruch in a review article in the New England Journal of Medicine recently, the more one consumes, the more oxidative stress our cells are under, and the more rapidly they perish. However, after the age of 75 a few extra pounds, particularly if it is muscle, is healthy.

According to a more recent article published in the Aug. 27, 1999, issue of *Science*, Drs. Weinbruch and Prella used a new technology of DNA microarrays. These are computer chip-like glass slides that have thousands of genes attached to them in a regular array or lay-out. Over 6,000 genes were represented and implanted in various tissues of mice and used as co-markers of aging. Of all the interventions, most of the life extension was by caloric restriction. The scientists concluded that a reduction of calories does impact on decreasing most hormone receptors actively and turn off whole blocks of genes. The Sir2 (silent information regulator no. 2) was discovered by a MIT research team. This is thought to influence the body just as caloric reduction (Imai et al *Nature*, 2000, 403:798-800). This directly influences the biologic aging of tissue and in general, the total organism. The Error and Repairs, Cross Linkage, Redundant DNA, Autoimmune, Order to Disorder, Gene Mutation, Rate of Living theories, all had some validity, but are now generally discarded.

## THE CLOCK-LIKE BODY

With my patients, I often compare the aging process to the clock. We are born with just so many tick-tocks embedded in our genes, or given to us by our Creator. As we get older, the clock winds down as all clocks wind down eventually — even a nuclear one. But, just like the spring-loaded clocks made in the last 400 years, we should work perfectly until the last several minutes, falter slightly — and then stop. We should have 100 years of prime living before the clock strikes OLD AGE. To continue the analogy of the clock, starting at age 20, when we reach adulthood, we cannot and should not turn the hands on the clock backwards, although it can be reset with knowledge of the proper bionutrient mechanics. The following paragraph will detail just how our nutritional neurobiological behavior can be optimized.

## PATHWAY TO LONGEVITY

We must stay out of harms way!!! One must physically, emotionally and psychologically stay out of risky situations. Stress leads to many ailments. In the New England Journal of Medicine (January 1997), Bruce McEachen, Ph.D., discusses the alostatic load. Allostasis is the ability to achieve stability through change, and is critical for a long survival. To some extent, the sudden secretion of adrenaline that prepares our body for fight or flight may be good for us if indeed we have to fight or flee. Our adrenal glands are activated by our pituitary to produce adrenaline and cortisol. In our society, conflict that has to be resolved psychically rather than physically, is dangerous. Since we are emotionally fighting, fleeing or frightening, we are literally abusing our bodies during an adrenaline rush with the extreme revving up of our engine, without muscular motion. This is likened to racing the engine of an automobile for hours while the gears remain in neutral and the car not moving. Any mechanic will tell you that this will wreck the engine. This stance without motion is causing spasms to our blood vessels and raising our cholesterol and adding stress to our engine-like heart. To add insult to injury, Dharma Singh Khalsa, M.D., relates in his recent book that our adrenals also release a massive amount of cortisol. This excessive cortisol causes irreversible injury to our vital organs including the heart, causing coagulation necrosis, death of neurons (brain cells) and senescence to our immune system. This may be the reason that the older we are, the more likely we are to have heart disease, dementia, cancer and overwhelming infections.

Cherishing the one you love will add 6.5 years to your life. A long term, committed relationship is achievable but as said, many times both partners need to give 100%. So if one spouse that moment gives nothing, the other will compensate by giving 100%. If you are in an unstable or unhappy relationship, get counseling to improve your situation. In the off chance that this does not work, when the children are raised (since you should be more committed to them than the spousal relationship for the sake of society) then break up. If a divorce is imminent, lean on loved ones, friends and counselors to minimize stress and needless aging.

Love your neighbor, hate no one. People who have lots of friends, social and particularly church support (see page 8 live longer and better. Loathing, holding a grudge, and thinking bad of ones fellow man or woman is taking years off your life. In the *Journal of the American Medical Association* article, May 17, 2000, cynical distrust and even more so hostility (Type H) caused ten times the risk of having abnormal coronaries in young adults. Get enough sleep by hook (naturally) or by crook (herbs, meditation, or a prescription drug). This is seven to eight hours a night or shorter with a daytime nap or meditation (see page 45). Having a pet, particularly a dog can extend ones life. Walk the dog. It's good for the pet and better for the owner. Do not be a risk taker. One must avoid circumstances that could be dangerous, such as driving too fast, not wearing a seatbelt, driving under the influence of drink or stress, taking chances by passing on the right, or not having enough clearance for left passage. You are twice as likely to be killed while walking with your back to traffic as when you face traffic says the National Safety Council. Occupying yourself with car phones or the radio/CD while driving is also dangerous. Accidents do take their toll in maimed or dead bodies. The survivability in a potentially fatal accident is ten times more in a big car (2,800 pounds or more) compared to a small automobile, according to Dr. Fred Rivara, a researcher at the University of Washington in Seattle. Smoke alarms should be installed in your home. While in a hotel, public building, or airplanes, know where the nearest emergency exit is, in case of a fire or other catastrophe. Do not go out alone in a strange or large city at night. Go easy in dangerous sports, such as mountain climbing. Do not ever over-drink alcoholic beverages or take mind-altering drugs. Do not have surgery unless there is no good alternative. Do not take any chances that may be dangerous unless it is a life or death emergency and the risk/benefit ratio is overwhelming on the benefit side. Be aware especially in poor lighting, of edges of carpets, thresholds of entrance ways, or misplaced objects in your path. I am sure you can think of many other examples of staying out of harms way and, of course, you also should know not to harm since in the big scheme of things, "what goes around, comes around."

## ARISTOTLE SAID IT

Moderation in all things, this golden rule, means nothing to excess. It should be your motto. Eating, drinking, exercising, playing and resting properly is necessary. We should consume the full (but not overdose) compliment of supplements such as vitamins and minerals. Try to stay as natural as possible. It is true, we do have a science in nutrition, but it is still in its infancy. There are yet many other vitamins and essential factors in the wings waiting to be discovered, and consumption of natural products will have these prime ingredients of life compared to synthetics or partial compounds we think today is healthy. Avoid toxin exposure, by staying away from pesticides, herbicides, chemicals in cleaning, paints and various aerosols as noted earlier in this chapter. Additionally, organic foods (see page 96) and unchlorinated water (see page 99 and yogurt (see page 93) should be used to maintain a healthy internal, compost pile. Good dress, fresh air, and exposure to proper light are also healthful. Having the appropriate metaphysical philosophy for the mind and spirit, as well as appropriate exercise, should be included in attaining a healthy lifestyle to insure longevity.

## WONDERFUL OXYGEN

When I discussed the oxygen sensitive Death Hormone Theory or DECO (see page 128) mention was made that oxygen could be a life extender. Live, work and play in an environment that is as free as possible from pollutants in the air. In the mountains, by the seashore, in the forest, or in small villages are best. A fresh supply of filtered air in your indoor environment is a must. There should be a good supply of oxygen in that air. Green plants indoors are helpful in that they take in carbon dioxide and manufacture oxygen. In our bodies, hemoglobin, which carries oxygen, sends a message to the blood vessel through which the red blood cell is coursing by releasing nitric oxide, which will increase even more the minute blood supply.

**Exercise with oxygen therapy** is espoused by Dr. William Campbell Douglas, who refers to this type of procedure as EWOT. Exercising while breathing concentrated oxygen, markedly increases the amount of oxygen in your blood plasma (that liquid which is left over when one takes the cells out of whole blood). It is that fluid which bathes our every cell. Extra oxygen will actually push more oxygen into our individual cells. Dr. von Ardenne's research in the late 1970's details more than 10,000 individual studies. He showed conclusively that there was a direct correlation between physical and psychological stress and blood oxygen levels. Perhaps too much of a good thing is bad and we physicians made too much of the subject of oxygen toxicity which, in my estimation, should be relegated to newborns and those patients who have been mismanaged by oxygen under pressure with devices we use in ventilation therapy. As we get older, we lose the ability to both, absorb and "burn" oxygen. By age 60, most of us have lost 40 percent of our ability to do this. Other factors, such as stressors (acute and chronic illness, surgery and extreme exercises) have the same effect and are additives to our aging process.

Getting started on the oxygen therapy may be as easy as joining a cardiac or a respiratory rehabilitation program where there is both oxygen and the needed exercise equipment. If this is not available, or if you do not have a heart disease or lung problem for which third party payers will pay for your treatment, you can finance it yourself and do it at home. It is not very expensive. Oxygen is a drug and one will need to have a doctor's prescription for it, but in this context it is safe and your doctor should accommodate you.

Again, with such diagnoses as heart failure, polycythemia and chronic lung disease with an oxygen saturation below 85 percent, your insurance should pay for it.

Although an oxygen concentrator may end up being cheaper and easier to maneuver in the long run and is easily rented from a durable medical goods supplier, some folks prefer the initially less expensive tank of oxygen rented and placed in the proper position by the local welding supply company. This 100 pound tank will last many weeks and the company will supply you with a gauge and a little tube to be placed around your nose. Recently, medical suppliers have made available tanks of liquid oxygen which they will dispense with a backpack oxygen bottle for portable use. You may have seen the unfortunate folks sitting in the doctor's office waiting room with these portable devices for their already ruined hearts or lungs. These are completely portable and can be used while jogging, bike riding, etc. Each of these tanks can last for three hours before refills are needed, which can be done from your own storage tank of liquid oxygen at home. They can be filled easily in less than four minutes.

Perhaps even better than oxygen is ozone, which is naturally made by the oxygen in the air if it is moving in abundant supply, such as by the ocean or on high peaks. Ozone is also made as lightning strikes the ground. It can also be synthesized by small electric currents, either intentionally in special machines or unintentionally in certain instances where electricity is energizing in the presence of oxygen. Devices costing less than $50 are available and there are practitioners that use ozone medically by placing it into living tissues such as blood or muscle. Breathing pure ozone, though, would be lung damaging. Do not confuse this ozone with the Ozone layer surrounding the earth which is thinning and causing the planet to gradually heat up by the "greenhouse effect." Be aware also of polluted air, such as smog or smaze, and that ozone may function negatively to make reactive molecules such as sulfuric and nitric acid.

Perhaps even better than EWOT or ozone therapy is hyperbaric (above normal pressure) oxygen therapy. Oxygen is normally delivered to tissues via the hemoglobin in your red blood cells; it is not dissolved in the liquid portion of your blood. However, in a pressurized environment, oxygen dissolves in all of the body's fluids: the plasma, the cerebrospinal fluid in the brain and spinal cord, and the lymph. It is then easily transported to all tissues, even those with a poor supply. When you breathe 100% oxygen in a hyperbaric oxygen chamber, virtually every cell of your body is flooded with a hundred times the amount of oxygen it normally gets.

Hyperbaric oxygen is administered in a specially designed chamber. Some chambers are made for one person in a reclining position and are filled with oxygen, while others hold several people. Pressure is slowly increased to 1.4 to 3 times that of the normal atmosphere. The typical treatment session lasts 45 minutes to two hours during which the patient relaxes in the chamber or listens to music. The pressure is then slowly returned to normal. Sessions may be repeated, depending on the condition, anywhere from five to 40 times. This therapy is fairly expensive and there is limit access with only 14 Medicare-approved uses. (Approved uses include serious skin and bone infections, carbon monoxide poisoning and skin grafts, not anti-aging). If money or third party payers were not an object, this remarkable regime should be given routinely, after age 40, and should be coupled with an alpha chamber. This is a contrivance in which a person lays and has the sensory application to put the body in a complete state of relaxation and the mind in the alpha carefree state.

## PROBIOTICS

Our intestines have been populated with friendly bacteria since day one of our birth. In our country, it is happenstance, that our bodies get the good bacteria from our mothers' germs and they indeed be the correct variety. In Germany this, not left up to chance, but drops of live bacteria cultures are given to newborns that will seed the colon appropriately and prevent a hostile flora (cultures of bacteria). Periodically to continue this healthy environment inside our intestines and prevent invasion and subsequent digestive problems, I recommend replanting our gut with probiotics.

Probiotics are a live culture of both bacteria and yeast. These are dedicated to not only discourage unfriendly organisms to take residence in our gut, but encourages good function of this organ. The proper pH, gas production, stool consistency, with a decreasing incidence of intestinal diseases is the result. These diseases include peptic ulcer (a hostile bacteria by the name of H. pylori) "colitis," gallbladder disease and cancer. The interest in probiotic use among the medical and scientific communities is shown by the fact that at least eight reviews in 2000 alone appeared in prestigious peer review journals devoted to microbiology in nutrition, and medicine.

The methodical scientific application of the probiotic concept to human health and disease is still in its infancy, but in my practice it has given excellent results. There are many commercial products available in health food stores and health catalogues. However, I recommend consuming live culture yogurt, which if one has a preparation, it can be used as a starter again and again for decades. Plain, low fat live cultured yogurt with acidophilus made by Dannon and other companies is used initially. With the last four tablespoons of this food, it is easy to add this to a quart of milk, placing this mixture warm oven for 6 to 8 hours will give a fantastic product. Also there are even easier methods to make this creation with a home yogurt maker. (See page 93 for other details).

In Germany and other industrial countries other than the U.S., the Bifidus organism is added. They also pay attention to the light spin of the bacterial product, making the beam rotate to the left or right, which is termed dextro (+) or levo (-). A mixture that produces both left and right turning molecules to light is called a racemic mixture. Since this is not ready for prime time in America, no need to worry about this concept. Yogurt itself contains two other organisms against unfriendly bacteria, along with the nice bacteria L-acidophilus and Bifidus. These will enhance our intestinal function by guarding us.

## UNCLE AL

A little like be a pro with probiotics, we can rapidly assess our nutritional status by the albumin level. A level less than 3.5 is indicative of malnutrition, says Dr. Stephen Sinatra, M.D., author of 16 books and editor of a well-read newsletter. Ken Seaton, Ph.D., an albumin expert, claims that this soluble protein is extremely versatile, playing a multifaceted role in our health. Albumin boosts the immune system, transports hormones, nutrients, vitamins, minerals, metals and amminoacids. Albumin aids in waste removal, cell growth, cell proliferation, cellular stability, electrolyte balance, kidney function, protein synthesis, immuno regulation and growth hormone activity. In 1992, the Journal of Science voted albumin as the Molecule of the Year. More recent research has shown albumin to liberate nitric oxide enhancing EDRF (Endothelium Derived Releasing Factor). This relaxes our arterial walls, prevents coronary artery spasm and figures importantly in preventing angina pectoris and myocardial infarction (chest pain and heart attack). This is truly Viagra for the heart. Albumin is also a mild antioxidant in itself and figures into the production of HDL cholesterol metabolism. This blood test is done routinely by your doctor in a chemistry profile.

## HOW TO EAT

Needless to say, we must eat healthily and properly. However, as we age, so does our gastrointestinal tract and we ingest fewer and fewer nutrients. The vicious cycle intensifies in that the less we absorb, the poorer our system works and even fewer nutrients are absorbed. Specifically, 30 percent of people over the age of 60 have less acid made by their stomachs than is normal. This inhibits the cascade of ensuing digestive enzymes in being released from this organ (pepsin) and the rest of the intestines (lipase, amylase, trypsin, chymotrypsin) as well as preventing the gallbladder from doing its thing by releasing the beneficial fat emulsifier, bile. To make matters worse, the intestines themselves do not transport food substances as actively and as well as they age. As a consequence, some older people literally die of malnutrition, they waste away. With poor nutrition, the immune system becomes incompetent and infections, some of which could be life-threatening, do occur. Eating slowly and comfortably in nice surroundings gives additional efficiency in the digestive process. Eating properly is necessary for normal albumin levels.

More than eating properly, more protein and vitamins and minerals need too be taken than when we were younger. Occasionally, we have indigestion, specifically bloating and gas, after eating, indicating decreased stomach acidity as noted earlier. This can be simply checked by swallowing a pill that transmits the acid condition of the stomach to a radio receiver placed on the abdomen. Since this originated at the University of Heidelberg, it is referred to as a Heidelberg Test. Insurance usually pays for this easy office procedure. If acid and/or enzymes are deficient, Betaine HCL (an acid) and/or enzymes (pepsin, lipase and protease) can be taken in varying amounts with meals. No prescription is needed for these. Plant based enzymes seem to work better than those "stolen" from animals. Eating raw vegetables and fruit also supply us with their natural enzyme.

Bulk is an important part of our food and is needed for proper transit time and good movement of the bowel. Fiber can be naturally obtained in many food stuffs, or it can be used in a fortified form such as soy, psillium seed or flaxseed (see page 63). To help bowel movements, I do recommend a more natural position in which we relieve ourselves. For less than $50, one can buy a device such as a *Wells Stepper* to place on the floor around the toilet so that a squatting position is maintained, just as our forefathers have done for hundreds of centuries; as is still done in the Orient, where there are far less hemorrhoidal problems, appendicitis, diverticulosis, or cancer of the colon. Remember, the end of the small intestine and the large intestine is our personal compost pile. For proper preparation of compost, we need quality material, to include food, enzyme and good fermentation. The latter is supplied by friendly bacteria. Antibiotic usage, knowingly or not, such as in meat, whose host were given these to produce better flesh kill the friendly bacteria in our intestines. Additionally, chlorinated water will also lower the bacterial count. As noted earlier in the chapter, one can repopulate our intestines with live culture yogurt or probiotics. Having the proper balance of intestinal flora, our internal plantation ensures against its invasion of yeast, bacteria and viruses. The combination of a good bacterial growth and the proper substrate of healthy fibrous foods produces essential vitamins, stimulates our entire digestive system and maintains our vital immune chemical and hormonal balance. See Chapter 3 for other information on food.

*Grow old with me! The best is yet to be! The last of life, for which the first was made. Our times are in his hands. Who sayeth, "A whole I plan, youth shows but half; trust God; see all and don't be afraid!"*

*— Robert Browning*
*(Rabbi Ben Ezra)*

# FIVE

# MATERIA MEDICA

## GENERAL

IN THE FOLLOWING, I included vitamins (see page 141, herbs (see page 182), minerals (see page 170), and supplements (see page 211). This is far from a complete list. Some entries I have gone into greater detail, reflecting the literature that is more recent or not as well known. The literature changes infrequently on vitamins and minerals, occasionally on herbs, and almost daily on the other supplements as proprietors rush to the new health scene for altruistic and economic reasons. There is little government control here compared to the prescribed drugs. This I feel is good for our society since the FDA (Federal Drug Administration) stifles medical research in the name of protection for its citizens. Although there may be some variance of the monthly cost, $ represents $10 or less, $$ represents $20 or less, $$$ represents $30 or less, and $$$$ represents $40 more or less. When no $, the cost is not known or not relevant.

## I. VITAMINS

Once upon a time, there may have been enough vitamins in our food so additions were not needed. This has changed drastically. Similar to minerals, these too have been leached from the soil. Then there is the change in diet to more refined and less natural food, lacking the vitamins (and similar molecules) as well as the minerals. It is easier to write about these one by one as an entity and to define a particular vitamin. Nevertheless, one must realize that each is a factor in the larger equation of health and can function only in conjunction with their complimentary biochemical partner, sometimes referred to as "co-factors." A vitamin is a substance essential for life that one cannot synthesize. These phytonutrients are plant-based organic substances that are needed to help us avoid diseases and function at our very best. When given in micro amounts, they protect us from "deficiency" diseases. However if given in pharmacological or even larger doses, sometimes referred to as industrial amounts they will treat certain diseases.

The term "vitamin" was coined mistakenly 75 years ago from the phrase "vital amines" from ammonia-producing substances. But we now know better. These are minute amounts of an organic catalyst that cannot be manufactured in the body and must be ingested. The naming system for vitamins is inadequate, and it will be changed one of these days. In general, they were classified alphabetically. The confusion was made worse because as more vitamins were discovered, they were subclassed such as $B_6$, $B_{12}$, $D_2$, or $D_3$. This poor classification leaves no room for vitamins discovered more recently such as Coenzyme $Q^{10}$, bioflavonoids and other phytonutrients.

RDA (Recommended Daily Allowance) is an overworked, misunderstood, overestimated, bureaucratic term that is close to worthless in modern concepts of nutrition. There was much ado by the news media after a flurry of research in high blood levels of homocysteine and its link to cardiovascular disease. In response to a public outcry, the government raised the RDA of folic acid from 200mg to 400mg a day. The dosage is given in two measurements. One is in avoipas weight, usually in milligrams. The other is units of activity (U or I.U.). These hearken back to the old biological assay of a vitamin. The research on these was done-in different countries and led to different kinds of units. In more recent years, consensus groups have come up with international units (I.U.) that combine the varying units from the different nations.

Natural production of vitamins is better, I think. But I have not taken a big stand on the question of natural versus synthetic production. As mentioned in an earlier chapter, natural products cause rotation of a light shined through the crystal material to the left rather than to the right. This is sometimes Levo- or Dextro-rotation or in a synthetic vitamin half to the right and half to the left. This is called a racemic mixture and does not exist in true nature. Nevertheless, other than some amino acids and perhaps yogurt, it seems to make little difference in our metabolism.

## Table 5-I.
## VITAMIN DOSAGE

The range of recommended daily amounts in a healthy person are:

Beta Carotene (Provitamin A*) ......... 20, 000 to 50,000IU
Vitamin A* ........................................... 5,000 to 10,000IU
Thiamin (B1) ..................................... 50 to 100mg
Riboflavin (B2).................................... 5 to 50mg
Niacin (B3)..................................... 25 to 3,000mg
Niacinamide (B3) ..................................... 150 to 1,500mg
Pantothenic acid (B5) ................................. 250 to 500mg
Pyridoxine (B6)..................................... 50 to 250mg
Vitamin $B_{12-}$ ..................................... 50 to 200mcg
Laetrile ($B_{17}$)..................................... 75 to 1000mg
Vitamin C ..................................... 1,000 to 12,000mg
Vitamin D* ..................................... 400IU to1,200IU
Vitamin E*..................................... 400 to 1,000IU
Vitamin F* ..................................... (see page 159)
Vitamin K* ..................................... 5 to 10mg
Folic Acid..................................... 400 to 1,200mcg
Bioflavonoids ..................................... 50 to 150mg
Biotin ..................................... 200 to 300 mcg
Choline..................................... 500 to 1,000mg
Inositol ..................................... 500 to 1,000mg
PABA..................................... 50 to 100mg

**\*Fat soluble**          **Others are water soluble**

## Properties of Vitamins

Generally, a water soluble vitamin "washes" out of our system in a day or two. But fat soluble vitamins will last months. The question of whether to take vitamins with food or without food is of minimal importance. Nevertheless, nature wanted us to get vitamins naturally as we ate. Therefore, it makes sense to take them in the proper amounts to supply the needs for your body's metabolism. Some vitamins are needed for the metabolism of food stuffs. Others fulfill an essential biochemical mechanism. Most vitamins have anti-oxidant activity. Fats, protein, carbohydrates are macronutrients, a storage form of energy. These are converted by the body into glucose, or simple blood sugar. The body "burns" glucose in the form of fuel in the presence of oxygen to produce carbon dioxide, water and an energized molecule. This oxidative process takes place in a microorgan in the cell called mitochondria. The energized chemical is a phosphated compound called ATP (Adenosine Triphosphate). This ATP is the electrical battery that powers our body. The by-product of this oxidative (chemical) reaction is the production of *free radicals.* These are molecules that are electrically unstable, containing an extra electron on their outer shell. The free radicals are useful in destroying bacteria and combating a variety of microdisease processes.

But when free radicals are not needed, however, they do mischief. They can attack our very own tissue such as the membranes around our cells to cause disease. If they attach to DNA, they can cause cancer. It can oxidize cholesterol to a particle that is rapidly taken in the blood vessel walls, causing atherosclerosis or, in lay terms, "hardening of the arteries." Free radicals cause at least 50 degenerative diseases including aging, Alzheimer's, Parkinson's disease, atherosclerosis and arthritis. These free radicals are neutralized or balanced with a system of antioxidant enzymes that include Glutathione, Catalase and Superoxide Desmutase (S.O.D.). These biochemicals and their pathways have been so ingeniously constructed that they are preserved or rejuvenated in the presence of antioxidant vitamins. The antioxidant trios of Vitamin C, E and Beta Carotene has been advocated for a long time as the most important combination in the treatment of degenerative diseases although in recent year, Beta Carotene has some bad press.

## $ Vitamin A

Vitamin A is a fat-soluble vitamin found in liver and in deep green, yellow or orange fruits. If not enough Vitamin A is taken, night blindness and ectodermal (skin and teeth) problems arise.

The RDA calls for 5,000 IU but larger amounts are needed to produce more health-giving tissues. For example, 50,000 IU a day may be used for treatment of leukolplakia, a white patch in the mouth, an early form of cancer. At least that amount is needed to prevent and treat viral infections such as measles and respiratory- syncytial virus. In addition, studies have shown that when there were abnormally low levels of the Vitamin in the blood (less than 45mcg%) there was a much higher incidence and mortality of HIV, Alzheimer's, cancer, heart disease and respiratory disease. Vitamin A should be used to help heal tissues under physical stress, such as surgery, infections, heart attack, and stroke.

There have been medical descriptions of Vitamin A toxicity. But I have never seen a case. Nor have any colleagues known to me. However, taking more than 20,000 IU a day should be under a knowledgeable doctor's supervision, to get the good from it without any harm.

## $ Vitamin $B_1$ (Thiamine)

$B_1$, a coenzyme, is a catalyst in the metabolism of carbohydrates and in enables simple sugars to release their energy. $B_1$ sources include leafy green vegetables, whole cereals, wheat germ, berries, nuts and legumes. In its natural state, rice is rich in $B_1$ but milling removes most of the vitamin. White flour and polished white rice are lacking in $B_1$. Rice husks, a byproduct of white rice, has much $B_1$ as well as other excellent micronutrients and are found in some commercial products. $B_1$ has a calming and focusing effect on the nervous system.

Even in today's world, we still see deficiencies in such diseases as alcoholism that produces abnormalities in thinking (Koraskov's Snydrome), seeing (Wernicke's Syndrome) and nerve conditions (Neuropathy). Although fewer than two milligrams a day are needed, diseases are treated with as much as 200mg at a time.

## $ Vitamin $B_2$ (Riboflavin)

Vitamin $B_2$ is a coenzyme that serves as a catalyst in fats, proteins and carbohydrates. Sources include dark, green vegetable, whole grain and mushrooms. It helps keep skin and mucous membranes healthy. An abundant supply results in youthful skin, particularly around the nose and mouth. Scandinavian research has shown it to have been used in dosages 400mg a day of to thwart migraine headaches or to ameliorate the symptoms of premenstrual syndrome. Nature sources include whole grains, cereals, avocados, green beans, spinach and bananas.

## $ Vitamin $B_3$
## (Niacin, Nicotinic Acid) (Nicotinamide, Niacinimide)

Found in lean meats, organ meats, fish, brewer's yeast, whole grains, nuts, dried peas and beans, white meat of turkey or chicken, milk and milk products. Take note, Niacin (nicotonic acid) is not exactly the same as niacinamide (nicotinamide). $B_3$ is known to assist enzymes to break down proteins, fats and carbohydrates into energy. Niacin lowers cholesterol, triglycerides and raises HDL cholesterol. It may help the nervous system and maintain healthy skin, tongue and digestive tissues. $B_3$ plays a role in the production of bile salts and for synthesis of sex hormones. Nicotinamide alleviates the pain of arthritis.

Severe deficiency results in Pellagra (which is rarely seen) that includes diarrhea and dementia, bright red tongue, sore tongue and gums, inflamed mouth, throat and esophagus, canker sores, mental illness, perceptual changes in the five senses, schizophrenic symptoms, rheumatoid arthritis, muscle weakness, general fatigue, irritability, recurring headaches, indigestion, nausea, vomiting, bad breath, insomnia, small ulcers. The RDA is 20mg. Niacin in doses of 1000 to 8000mg a day, lowers cholesterol. Nicotinamide in similar amounts does combat the pain in muscular skeletal diseases.

Although non prescription, there are significant effects. Almost all will get a flushing 30 to 90 minutes after taking crystalline niacin. Isohexoniacinate (IHN) and the slow release product does not cause this nuisance side effect. Taking small doses of 10-25 mg daily and gradually increasing will initiate this annoying symptom. More worrisome is the elevation of blood sugar, liver dysfunction, peptic ulceration, increases of uric acid, eye problems, and skin infections. In doses of more than 1000 mg a day, periodic monitoring by a knowledgeable physician is recommended. A prescription of a long acting niacin, Niaspan has been available since 1997.

$B_3$, particularly nicatinamide, may increase our life span in a way similar to continued caloric restriction. $B_3$ makes up much of NAD (nicotinamide adenine dinucleotide) used by our cells for energy production when other sources are low. Eating minimal for the rest of our lives means less energy production, less wear and tear and most importantly, less oxidative damage from the energy production research MIT has isolated the gene Sir2 (for *silent regulation no.2*) and its protein Sir2p. In many lower species, turning on of this gene greatly increases its life span by working through NAD. The more the NAD, the better Sir2p functions. NADH is available as a supplement (used for chronic fatigue syndrome, see page 253), but does not promote any significant levels of Sir2p. Nicotinamide 500-1000 mg a day is recommended to treat the pain of arthritis anywhere from 500-5000 mg a day are needed. Beware in high doses as noted above, there are side effects.

## $ Vitamin $B_5$ (Panothenic acid, Calcium Pantothenate,Panthenol)

Found in brewer's yeast, liver, kidney, wheat bran, crude

molasses, whole grains, egg yolk, peanuts, peas, sunflower seeds, beef, chicken, turkey, milk and royal jelly, $B_5$ is vital for the adrenal glands and for production of cortisone. It plays a role in creating energy from protein, carbohydrates and fats helping to synthesize cholesterol, steroids and fatty acids. Used for a healthy digestive tract and essential to production of antibodies, it will help with arthritis and is an anti-inflammatory.

The deficiency symptoms are a burning sensation in the feet; enlarged beefy, tongue; duodenal ulcers, inflammation of the intestines and stomach; decreased antibody formation; upper respiratory infections; vomiting; restlessness; muscle cramps; constipation; adrenal exhaustion; overwhelming fatigue; reduced production of hydrochloric acid in the stomach; allergies; arthritis; nerve degeneration; spinal curvature; disturbed pulse rate; gout; graying hair. The optimal daily amount: 100-200mg in a B-complex supplement or up to 500mg in divided doses. RDA is 10mg. Many nutritionists feel that B vitamins should be given with each other, not to cause a relative deficiency. I personally have seen no problems by giving just one at a time.

### $ Vitamin $B_6$ (Pyridoxine, Pyridoxinal, Pyridoxamine)

Found in brewer's yeast, sunflower seeds, wheat germ, liver and other organ meats, blackstrap molasses, bananas, walnuts, roasted peanuts, canned tuna and salmon, $B_6$ metabolizes proteins, fats and carbohydrates; it forms hormones for adrenaline and insulin and makes antibodies and red blood cells. It is used for synthesis of RNA and DNA; regulates fluids in the body and is needed for production of hydrochloric acid. It can relieve carpal tunnel syndrome, fluid retention, PMS symptoms, helps asthmatics, and when used with magnesium, helps prevent kidney stones.

The deficiency symptoms are greasy, scaly skin between the eyebrows and on the body parts that rub together; low blood sugar; numbness and tingling in the hands and feet; neuritis; arthritis; trembling hands in the aged; water retention and swelling during pregnancy; nausea; motion sickness; mental retardation; epilepsy; kidney stones; anemia; excessive fatigue; nervous breakdown; mental illness; acne; convulsions; babies and newborn infants may develop crusty yellow scabs on the scalp called "cradle cap." The optimal daily amount is 50-100mg (combined with a B-complex supplement). RDA is 2mg. This is part of the Vitamins Triad ($B_6$, $B_{12}$, and Folic Acid) is to prevent and treat homocystemia.

## $ Vitamin $B_{12}$ (Cyanocobalamine)

$B_{12}$ is necessary in small amounts for the formation of proteins, red blood cells, maintenance of the inner lining of the intestinal tract and for the function of the central nervous system. In the latter instance, it produces myelin the material that serves as insulation for the "wires" of the brain, spinal cord and peripheral nerves. $B_{12}$ is not available from vegetable sources. It is produced only by microbes - bacteria and algae. Microbes found in the mouth and intestines produce enough $B_{12}$ for most of us. Because of the introduction of antibiotics, it has become possible, though highly unlikely, that a strict vegetarian can produce deficiency. The problem is that $B_{12}$ is an unusual vitamin in that it needs a helper, a special substance called "Intrinsic Factor," to activate it so it can be absorbed in the end of the ileum, (the small intestine immediately before the large intestine or colon).

A number of reasons can lead to deficiency: We do not consume enough of it in our food. The stomach doesn't produce the Intrinsic Factor and/or hydrochloric acid because it has been removed surgically or has been 'poisoned' by drugs used by doctors and as we get older, it just naturally decreases. Also, the end of our small intestine has been removed surgically, just doesn't function well or has been damaged by disease or radiation. Pernicious anemia is the result of inadequate $B_{12}$. Raw liver protects people from this disease — a discovery that led to the Nobel Prize for George Whipple and George Murphy in 1934. Even if there is a slight deficiency, there is a build up of homocysteine. Homocysteine, a natural body chemical, if elevated is as deadly as sky-high cholesterol. Besides the question of the quantity of $B_{12}$. there is also one resulting from a low $B_{12}$ carrying protein. Some patients also have a partial blockage in getting it into the brain and need much higher levels than the 200-1200 picograms. This deficiency may be part of the CFS/Fibromyalgia syndrome (see page 253).

In the past, doctors used $B_{12}$ injections for a myriad of diseases and they did, indeed, help the patient feel better. However, once patients obtained levels thought to be normal and insurance companies refused to pay for injections, many new doctors unwittingly deprived patients of this needed vitamin. For at least 50 years, experienced practitioners knew that a symptomatic improvement of well-being occurred with a regular injection, of $B_{12}$. Some nutritionally oriented physicians have discovered that 1,000mcg (1 mg) a day abolishes asthma and is helpful in many other conditions, such as Alzheimer's disease, chronic fatigue syndrome, and many neurological disorders. These patients actually have a functional deficiency of the vitamin. Once they have an abundance, their diseases are improved or even cured.

There now is a test for this functional deficiency, in the presence of adequate blood levels, where an oral dose of homocysteine and methylmalonic acid are given and the blood is tested for the production of L-methionine. The dose of $B_{12}$ is variable. I usually recommend 1,000mcg injections a month, 1,000 mcg orally, 2mg daily taken under the tongue or as a nasal gel to bypass the stomach. The stomach may not have been making enough Intrinsic Factor or the small intestine may be impaired and not absorbing well, so a super large dose is given. Vitamin $B_{12}$ is extremely safe with the only downside being a slight case of acne if too much is given too often. The best forms are hydroxycobalamine or methyl cobalamine compounded by a pharmacist compared to the cyanocobalamine, which is by prescription commercially available for injectible use. In theory, too much cyanocobalamine could cause cyanide toxicity. As much as

20,000U a day for 10 years by injection has been given with apparently no side effects.

### Vitamin B$_{13}$ (Orotic Acid)

Actually, there is not much information about orotic acid. It has been used recently as orotate salts combined with such minerals as calcium, magnesium, and potassium. This is based on the work by German doctor the late Hans Nieper. Dr. Nieper's work has included treatment of multiple sclerosis and other chronic diseases with these mineral orotates. His experience concluded that orotate salts were active transporters of these minerals into the blood from the gastrointestinal tract. The salts then separate from the mineral in the blood, allowing the mineral to be used and leaving orotic acid available.

Orotic acid is found in a few natural food sources-for example, milk products and some root vegetables, such as carrots, beets, and Jerusalem artichokes. Orotic acid is a nucleic acid precursor and is needed for DNA and RNA synthesis. The body can make orotic acid for this purpose from its amino acid pool. As long as protein nutrition is adequate, the body can carry on nucleic acid synthesis. Neither toxicity or deficiency of orotic acid are likely a concern.

Recently, many medical claims for orotates have been made by foreign markets and the U.S. health industry. Due to this reason and possibly other political-economic ones, the U.S. Food and Drug Administration (FDA) has asked for the removal of orotates from the U.S. marketplace.

### Vitamin B$_{15}$ (Pangamic Acid)

This is still a fairly controversial "vitamin." The quotation marks suggest that we are not sure whether it is a vitamin. It has not yet been shown to be essential in the diet (vitamins must be supplied from external sources), and no symptoms or deficiency diseases are clearly revealed when consumption is restricted. The FDA has been concerned about the wide range of medical conditions treated with it, primarily in other countries, and therefore pangamic acid is not readily available to the U.S. consumer. Because most of the information about pangamic acid is dated and is mainly from European and Soviet research, I discuss this substance here mainly for completeness.

Pangamic acid is found in kernels and whole grains such as brown rice, brewer's yeast, pumpkin and sunflower seeds, and beef blood. Water and direct sunlight may reduce the potency and availability of $B_{15}$ in these foods.

Pangamic acid is mainly a methyl donor, which helps in the formation of certain amino acids such as methionine. It may play a role in the oxidation of glucose and in cell respiration. By this function it may reduce hypoxia (deficient oxygen) in cardiac and other muscles. Like vitamin E, it acts as an antioxidant, helping to lengthen cell life through its protection from oxidation. Pangamic acid is also thought to offer mild stimulation to the endocrine and nervous systems, and by enhancing liver function, it may help in the detoxification process. As a methyl donor, SAMe is far better and more available. There is no known toxicity or deficiency of Vitamin $B_{15}$.

There is limited information about deficiencies of pangamic acid. There are no clear problems when it is absent in the diet, though some diminished circulatory and oxygenation functions are possible. Decreased cell respiration-that is, decreased oxygen use by cells may influence many other cellular functions which may lead to negative effects on the heart.

There is no RDA for pangamic acid. At the time of this writing, it is not legal to distribute $B_{15}$ in the United States, though it was used as a supplement for some time in the 1970s. The most common form of pangamic acid was calcium pangamate, but currently it is dimethyl glycine (DMG), which may even be the active component that has been hailed in the Soviet Union. Pangamic acid or DMG, when used, is often taken with vitamin E and vitamin A. A common amount of DMG is 50-100 mg. taken twice daily, usually with breakfast and dinner. This level of intake may improve general energy levels, lowers homocysteine, support the immune system, and is also thought to reduce cravings for alcohol and thus may be very helpful in moderating chronic alcohol problems.

### $$$$ Vitamin B$_{17}$ (Laetrile Amygdaline)

Laetrile was discovered by Dr. Ernest Krebs, a Nobel prize winner for the glucose metabolism pathway named for him (Krebs cycle). He initially thought that this was a vitamin and wrote about its virtues. The proponents of laetrile claim that it is a natural molecule found in food and is not toxic in normal doses and should not be under FDA control. This is the controversial drug that has been used for cancer but banned from this country in the '70s. This vitamin contains thiocyanate and is intimately involved with over a score of major body functions. Thiocyanate, be it either deficit or too much, has an adverse effect on body metabolism. Thiocyanate is found mostly in nuts, particularly the apricot kernel. In the 1940s, B$_{17}$ was used to treat rheumatism and hypertension. Another drug, nitroprusside, with a cyanate is used as a temporary treatment of overwhelming hypertension and heart failure today.

Because of toxicity concerns, the dose of B$_{17}$ is limited to one gram daily. A blood serum, thiocyanate (BST) is obtained. BST level is monitored and kept between four and seven percent. Natural sources of this vitamin can be obtained by eating ten to twenty apricot kernels a days. These are blended or pulverized and consumed immediately. One to two cups of fresh mung bean sprouts may provide an equivalent amount. Laetrile changes thyroid metabolism and it alters the TSH. It releases thyroxin from the albumin and initially causes an increase of thyroid and subsequently a decrease. This may be needed in certain states of "sick thyroid syndrome" in which the patient with a variety of bad diseases is noted to have a depressed thyroid because of that illness. Laetrile is available in over thirty countries. Many U.S. patients with cancer go to Mexico for their supply.

## $ Vitamin C

Vitamin C is the most widely used vitamin. It also is called ascorbic acid, since it was the agent used to prevent scurvy in the 16th century. The vitamin is found naturally in fruits, partially citrus, and vegetables. Its water solubility also means that excessive amounts are eliminated through urination. Evolution has deprived humans of the ability to produce vitamin C but most other animals do manufacture it for their own bodies. The RDA is 60 mg-an amount designed to prevent scurvy. One-tenth of an orange a day or one fifth of a lime will prevent the dreaded disease of old-time sailors (limeys), alcoholics and individuals with odd diets. In 35 years as a clinician, I have seen only one case of scurvy. The dose depends on the purpose. It helps repair tissue. So higher doses may be needed following surgery and other physical and emotional diseases to which we can fall prey. I recommend at least one gram (1,000 mg) a day. But if you are under stress of disease or surgery, I would recommend two to three grams a day. Some colleagues give two grams every hour until explosive diarrhea occurs. For an acute cold, it is not unusual for people to take six to eight grams a day. The scientist, Linus Pauling, took 18 grams a day for decades and lived to be 94. Pauling won the Nobel Prize for the discovery of the true importance of vitamin C.

Research has shown postitive results in its role of preventing heart disease, cancer, some infections, birth defects, and aging. Because it is water soluble, some experts advise taking half the daily amount twice a day. In rare instances, higher doses can cause gastrointestinal problems, such as diabetes. Reducing the dose will stop diarrhea. The upper gastrointestinal problems can be stopped by reducing the dose to less than one gram a day, taking the dose with food, or better yet, taking Ester-C. It seems if one has a problem that really is vitamin C responsive, such as a viral infection, the dose can be easily increased to 20-40 grams a day without any diarrhea, but when the infection resolves this dose then would cause diarrhea.

## $ Vitamin D

Vitamin D is misunderstood by most physicians. Most of us know of it as the "sunshine vitamin." It prevents rickets. High doses of this fat-soluble vitamin is toxic, but vitamin D isn't really a vitamin. It has long been classified as a vitamin because our bodies cannot manufacture it and it must be obtained from outside sources. However, we do make and absorb vitamin D from our skin. In the body, vitamin D behaves like a hormone, interacting with parathyroid hormone to control calcium balance. It is required for the absorption of calcium from the intestines and into the bones. This explains its role in preventing rickets, a childhood disease of softened, misshapen bones caused by inadequate calcium in the bone, as well as osteomalacia, the adult counterpart of rickets, and osteoporosis. See Chapter Seven, page 289.

Since these consequences of vitamin D deficiencies-and their cure with vitamin D-rich cod-liver oil-were discovered 75 years ago, these once common disorders have virtually disappeared. An unfortunate result of this, however, is the lingering misconception that vitamin D deficiency is exclusively linked with these conditions. Although rickets may be a thing of the past, vitamin D deficiencies are still with us. The 21st century vitamin D deficiency disease is not rickets but osteoporosis. Also associated with vitamin D deficiencies are higher rates of cancer of the breast, ovary, prostate, colon and rectum; increased incidence of multiple sclerosis; progression of osteoarthritis, impaired immune response, hypertension, and mood disorders.

It has long been known that certain groups are at risk of vitamin D deficiencies: residents of nursing homes; people over 65, especially those who are housebound; and individuals living in northern latitudes, particularly during the winter. This is because the body's synthesis of this fat-soluble vitamin is dependent upon exposure to sunlight. Ultraviolet radiation prompts the conversion of cholesterol, a vitamin D precursor in the skin, which is further altered in the liver and kidneys to become the active forms of this hormone-like vitamin.

In reality, we are all at risk of vitamin D deficiency, as a 1998 study carried out at Massachusetts General Hospital clearly showed. Fifty-seven percent of all patients admitted to the hospital were vitamin D deficient. These were not nursing home residents or elderly people. They represented the general population. Even more alarming, 37 percent of those who consumed the recommended daily allowance of vitamin D in food or supplements had low blood levels of 25 hydroxyvitamin D, or 25(OH)D, a reliable blood marker of vitamin D status.

The number one contributor to low vitamin D levels is decreased sun exposure, and Americans have made it a mission to avoid the sun. Today, however, the only parts of the body exposed to the sun on many people are their hands and face, which are often protected by sunscreen anyway. The limited exposure is simply not enough to generate adequate amounts of vitamin D. One needs to get out in the sun, without sunscreen or long sleeves (weather permitting), for 20 minutes at least three times a week. If your skin is dark and you are older than 65, try to soak up at least 40 minutes of sun, as your production of vitamin D is slower. (If you plan to be in the sun for prolonged periods, particularly in the summertime, I recommend using a sunscreen.) Your body does store some of this vitamin in fatty tissues for use during the winter, but as these widespread deficiencies attest, it's important to augment those stores.

A vitamin D supplement is much needed. One can get vitamin D from the diet. However, the only significant natural dietary contributor of vitamin D is fish oil. Dairy (excluding most yogurt and cheese products) and eggs contain a little, and fortified milk and cereal provide considerably more. Yet even with a healthy diet, few people consume more than 200 IU per day. If we are not getting enough sun exposure, and also not getting enough vitamin D in our diet, there's only one solution, take vitamin D supplements. The current daily recommended intake (DRI, the new version of the more familiar RDAs) of vitamin D for most adults is 200 IU, for those over 50 years of age 400 IU, and for the 70+

age group 600 IU. This may be enough to prevent rickets, but not osteopenia or osteoporosis. Additionally, a study shows that milk has a variable amount of vitamin D, 50 IU, and 850 IU per quart in others. In a well-documentd research paper in the May 1999 issue of the *American Journal of Clinical Nutrition*, Dr. Reinhold Vieth of the University of Toronto contends that the current DRIs are woefully inadequate and makes a strong case for a DRI of 800-1,000 IU per day.

Most of the propaganda concerning vitamin D's potential toxicity is overblown. Although alarmists warn of toxicity with as little as 1,000 IU per day, according to Dr. Vieth, "consistently literature to support (statements about the toxicity of moderate doses of vitamin D) has been either inappropriate or without substance." Some studies have administered 100,000 IU per day for brief periods with no adverse effects, and in one Finnish study, a 300,000 IU injection in the autumn safely lowered the incidence of osteoporotic fractures by 25 percent.

Try to get 20-40 minutes of unfiltered sun exposure at least three days a week, year-round, and to supplement with 800-1000 IU vitamin D. Most multivitamins contain 200-400 IU of vitamin D. I recommending augmenting that with an additional 400-600 IU. This is especially important during the winter and if one does not get adequate sun exposure. No prescription is needed for preparations less than 1000U. I frequently prescribe Vitamin D 50,000 weekly for patients without osteoporosis for over a decade and have had a good response without any toxicity.

### $ Vitamin E

Vitamin E, also called "B tocopherol," is a fat-soluble vitamin found in grains, nuts, oils and leafy green vegetables. This vitamin impacts the body with array of benefits ranging from sexual function in males to minimizing damage in a heart attack. I take 1,000 IU a day. I recommend between 400 and 1,200 IU a day. I have been told that it can cause a bleeding disorder in extremely doses higher than 6,000 IU.

But I have never seen a single case. Most formulations are given in denominations of an I.U. (International Unit). One International Unit is equal to one milligram; so it follows that 1,000 IU is equal to 1,000 mg.

There are several varieties of this molecule. Vitamin E actually is a nutrient complex with eight active components. Science has emphasized the four tocopherols. The most active one, alpha-tocopherol, is a well-established antioxidant. The synthesized version is what most people take as a Vitamin E supplement. The isolation of one active ingredient means missing out on something else. The other three tocopherols (beta, gamma and delta) are required, for each carries a corresponding chemical component called a tocotrienol. The average supplement consumer is unaware that toctrienols are individually stronger than their tocopherol partners. The entire nutrient complex is stronger still. As recent lab experiments demonstrate, the combined force of alpha, gamma and delta toctrienols can inhibit malignancy. Don't be surprised to see Vitamin E added to many more creams and cosmetics. Topical tocotrienols are being researched for their ability to protect the skin from the oxidative damage of ultraviolet radiation.

The main source of Vitamin E now is palm oil, though research has tested toctrienol supplements from barley. Soon these should be available as capsules of concentrate. Natural Vitamin E (d-alpha tocopherol) may be far better than the synthetic variety (dl-alpha tocopherol) in that it is much more compatible with liver tissue. Vitamin E, as a long-lasting antioxidant, may protect and even diminish such diseases that are oxidatively produced due to excess free radicals in chronic diseases such as atherolsclerosis, Alzheimer's, ulcerative colitis and restless leg syndrome. It also has been shown to minimize damage if given early in acute disease processes such as a heart attack. Vitamin E protects the oxidation of Vitamin A and fat. It neutralized LDL (Low Density Lipoprotein), also know as "bad cholesterol," and prevents its oxidation, the major cause of damage directly to the walls of our arteries. An abundance of Vitamin E is important for maximum sexual function particularly in men. Vitamin C helps to keep vitamin E working better and usually is given in conjunction with it. The U.S. daily diet is less than the recommended daily value (RDV) of 30 IU a day. Inorganic iron destroys vitamin E, but not the organic iron found in iron rich foods such as spinach and raisins.

## $$ Vitamin F (Essential Fatty Acids — EFA)

The unsaturated or essential fatty acids in our diet come primarily from liquid vegetable oils and fish. Commercial products of these contain vitamin E as well, which protects them from oxidation. There are two essential fatty acids which the body does not make and thus must be obtained from the diet. These are linoleic (LA) and linolenic (LNA) acids, found mainly in seeds, wheat germ, cod liver oil, and the golden vegetable oils, such as soy, safflower, and corn. Flaxseed oil is probably our best oil, being particularly high in both omega-3 as alpha-linolenic acid and omega-6 fatty acids in the right balance for us. Evening primrose oil is high specifically in gamma-linolenic acid, an omega-6 fatty acid, and the fish oils are high in omega-3 fatty acids, particularly eicosapentaenoic acid (EPA).

Linoleic acid is need for our body to make prostaglandin (a hormone-like substance — PG) of the E and $E_2$ which in the right proportion (1:2) to the $E_3$ series may be healthful. Linolenic, the precursor to $E_3$ has various effects on both smooth muscle and platelets (the small elements in the blood, causing clotting and inflammation). $E_3$ (PG $E_3$) causes a decrease in cholesterol, clotting and inflammation.

Deficiency of the EFAs can reduce growth and skin, tissue, and joint lubrication. Low levels in the body have been seen in such conditions as prostate enlargement, psoriasis, anorexia nervosa, hyperactivity, and multiple sclerosis. Deficiency problems of EFAs may include acne, diarrhea, dry skin, eczema, alopecia (hair loss), gallstones, and slow growth and wound healing.

Vitamin F has been used in the treatment of eczema, psoriasis, skin allergies, prostatitis, and asthma. It is required in amounts equaling at least 2 percent of caloric intake, 1-2 teaspoons a day depending on weight. (The essential fatty acids are discussed in more detail in Chapter 3.)

### $ Vitamin K (K, K₂, Menaquinone, Phytonadione)

Vitamin K is antiaging. Not only does it protect the blood vessels from atherosclerosis, but it also prevents osteoporosis, Alzheimer's disease, and cancer. Low vitamin K levels may also figure into diabetes. It is a powerful antioxidant and is a natural chelater with its action similar to the EDTA used in intravenous chelation therapy. Vitamin K works by regulating calcium. Bones need this, but arteries can't stand it. Vitamin K accommodates both of these organ systems. It's initial discovery, though was in coagulation, labeled vitamin K for the Danish work, Koagulation. Most folks erroneously feel it works only here.

Vitamin K works through an amino acid called "Gla," which stands for Gamma-carboxyglutamic acid. Gla is part of a specific protein that controls calcium. Fifteen such proteins have been found so far; and researchers believe there are at least one hundred scattered throughout the body. Vitamin K is the only vitamin that makes these proteins work. Vitamin K performs a feat on the proteins called "carboxylation." Carboxylation gives the proteins claws so they can hold onto calcium. Once the protein grabs onto calcium it can be moved around the body. Proteins that don't get enough vitamin K don't have the claws. They're "undercarboxylated" and can't control the mineral. Without a functioning protein to control it, calcium drifts out of bone and into arteries and other soft tissue. The calcium is frequently a marker for sick tissue on that it is deposited there because of the malfunction of Gla there.

The most famous Gla protein is "osteocalcin." You may have heard of osteocalcin in connection with bone density. What you might not have heard is that it requires vitamin K to work. Undercarboxylated osteocalcin (osteocalcin without vitamin K) can't regulate calcium. When this happens, calcium leaves bone and teeth. Women with "undercarboxylated osteocalcin" excrete calcium, and their bones are porous. Vitamin K reverses this trend. Vitamin K works with vitamin D. Vitamin D plays several roles in bone. One of them is provoking the osteocalcin gene into action. Once synthesized, however, osteocalcin needs vitamin K to function properly.

Osteoporosis may reflect serious health problems. If the 1993, updated in 1999 *Study of Osteoporotic Fractures* is correct, bone density is a striking predictor of death. In its first report, every standard deviation from normal bone density equaled a 20% greater risk of mortality in women age 65 or older. Therefore, two deviations from normal bone density equals a 40% greater risk of mortality, according to this study. People with osteoporosis did not die from broken bones, or complications from such bones. In fact, falling accounted for only 3% of the mortalities in this osteoporosis study. They died, instead, from heart attack, cancer and stroke. Why? The answer is beginning to be worked out.

One of the substances that age upregulates is Interleukin-6 (IL-6). IL-6 is a cytokine, a biochemical messenger for the immune system. In the aging body, IL-6 increases at the expense of other cytokines. This imbalance in the system creates inflammation. IL-6 has been discovered in arthritic joints and diseased blood vessels. In a striking study done at the National Research Institute in Italy, people with the highest amount of IL-6 were almost twice as likely to become physically immobile because of musculoskeletal problems and mentally immobile because of Alzheimer's Disease (AD). Vitamin K inhibits IL-6 and inflammation and perhaps the cause of both of these maladies.

We have known for almost two decades of apolipoprotein E and its relationship AD These are eight genetic types with E4 form connected to Alzheimer's Disease. They also have lower vitamin K levels. Dr. Martin Kohlmeier of the University of North Carolina believes it's no coincidence. He thinks there's a connection between the lack of vitamin K, apoE4 and the ability to regulate calcium in the brain. This is related to osteocalcin. It's one of the calcium-grabbing proteins in bone. But bone is not its only location. It's also found in the brain, along with other vitamin K-dependent proteins. People with the E4 protein have undercarboxylated osteocalcin not only in their bone, but also in their brains. Kohlmeier believes that people with E4 clear vitamin K too fast from their bodies. This leaves too little vitamin K for the brain proteins. Calcium can't be regulated properly and may cause some of the damage seen in AD. Studies show that AD patients have severely dysregulated calcium in their brains. This has to do with their lack of vitamin K-the vitamin necessary for controlling calcium in both the brain and bone. These people with E4 are also more prone to develop other "metal toxicities" such as lead and mercury because of lack of this natural chelator.

The pancreas has the second highest amount of vitamin K in the body. This suggests the vitamin may have something to do with controlling blood sugar. In the first study of its kind, researchers in Japan looked at vitamin K's effect on glucose and insulin. In a study on rats, they found that vitamin K deficiency initially impedes the clearance of glucose, then causes too much insulin to be released. This can be plotted on a graph that looks very similar to what occurs in diabetes in humans.

Some studies show that vitamin K is more powerful than vitamin E and coenzyme Q10 for scavenging free radicals. In a study on animals subjected to oxidative stress, vitamin K by itself completely protected the liver from free radicals (but not muscles). In another study, vitamin K was 80% as effective as vitamin E in preventing the oxidation of linoleic acid (a polyunsaturated fatty acid). According to researchers in the Netherlands, warfarin (a blood thinner) abolishes the antioxidant effect of vitamin K. Vitamin E and glutathione protect vitamin K's antioxidant effect.

Anticoagulant drugs work by interfering with vitamin K. Therefore, people taking "blood thinners" such as warfarin or heparin should not take vitamin K. People who chronically take these drugs are, in effect, vitamin K deficient. These people show effects on bone and blood vessels.

Studies show that long-term anticoagulant users have osteoporsis and a tendency to hemorrhage.

Vitamin K may prevent blood clots. Those taking ginkgo, aspirin, garlic or ginger to prevent blood clots and increase blood flow needn't worry that vitamin K will undo the effects. Vitamin K also prevents blood clots! It works by preventing "platelet aggregation," a process that is different from coagulation. Aggregation has to do with oxidative stress and free radicals, whereas coagulation is about the calcium level in cells. Vitamin K gets away with its dual personality because blood aggregation is different from coagulation. Vitamin K also plays a role in activating two factors that reverse clotting: proteins S and C. Studies show that people who have a deficiency of protein S and C get blood clots.

Green leafy vegetables supply 40-50% of vitamin K as noted on the next page. Vegetable oils are the next highest source. Hydrogenated oils (margarine, for example) create an unnatural form of K that may actually stop the vitamin from working and could cause relative vitamin K deficiency. There are three different types of vitamin K: K1 which is from plants, K2 which is made by bacteria and K3 which is synthetic. Vitamin K3 is generally regarded as toxic because it generates free radicals. However, this version shows promise in the treatment of some cancers. K2 specifically keeps calcium and phosphorus out of the aorta, and reverses the effects of heart-unfriendly diets. The body converts K1 to K2.

Vitamin K Stressors and osteoporosis should be the deciding factors to consider in taking this supplement. Antibiotics wipe out intestinal flora, which are the source of vitamin K2. Cholesterol-reducing drugs, low-fat diets, Olestra, and anything else that interferes with fat reduces vitamin K. Vitamin K is carted around the body by lipoproteins, the same proteins that carry cholesterol. In order for vitamin K to be absorbed, there must be some fat present. Mineral oil laxatives interfere with the absorption of vitamin K. Some hydrogenated oil, antibiotics, the food preservatives inhibit with the ability of vitamin K to function. Gastrointestinal diseases, gallstones, synthetic estrogens, liver malfunction, and anything else that interferes with the gut or bile can cause vitamin K deficiency. Dietary restriction or dieting also do this. Don't forget that dietary restriction only enhances longevity if all nutrients are maintained at high levels. And watch out for low-fat diets. It's the oil in the salad dressing that enables the vitamin K in your salad to be absorbed. Also be careful about diets such as high-protein meat diets that are devoid of green vegetables. (They also contain methionine, which raises the homcysteine). Hydrogenated, transaturated, polyunsaturated oils use in much commercial products and in home cooking decrease vitamin K's function. Warfarin (Coumadin) also reduces vitamin K, but most times the benefits from this anticoagulant outweigh the risks.

Food is the natural source of Vitamin K. The classic thinking is that vitamin K is only found in green leafy vegetables since it requires chlorophyll to be synthesized in plants. But plants store vitamin K in their fruits and seeds as well. Soy is an excellent source of vitamin K. Fermented products, including some cheeses, also contain vitamin K; their bacteria synthesize the vitamin. Spinach contains a special form of vitamin K that hasn't been found in any other vegetable. Plants today have far less vitamin K than decades ago due to environmental change and the fact that our soils do not have the nutrients that they have had in the past. Although fat soluble, vitamin K is not stored in the body, and is therefore nontoxic in high amounts. Forty-five milligrams a day were used in osteoporosis studies without any ill effect. Vitamin K has been approved in Japan for the treatment of osteoporosis since 1995. Several thousand times more than what people are currnetly getting in their diet has been taken without any toxicity. Dosage depends on an individual's diet, age, whether they are taking drugs, and what stressors are present. Generally, 10mg/day is recommended. If you want to get your vitamin K level tested, request the osteocalcin test. It is much more reliable than coagulation tests. The osteocalcin test measures how much carboxylated osteocalcin you have. Since carboxylation is dependent on vitamin K, this test will give you a good idea of your vitamin K status, and whether or not you're headed for premature degenerative disease and an earlier death.

## $ Folic Acid (Folacin or Vitamin M)

Folic acid is a coenzyme needed for forming protein and hemoglobin. It is available from green vegetables, whole grains and brewer's yeast. The best natural source is a fresh green garden salad. Unlike the other water soluble vitamins, folic acid can be stored in the liver so you do not need to eat it everyday. It is considered a B vitamin and acts like its cousins, B6 and B12 in that a deficiency figures into the homocysteine that causes premature atherosclerosis.

If the body doesn't have enough of it during pregnancy, congenital neurological birth defects are frequent. In high doses of 5mg a day, it is used to treat otherwise refractory arthritis and pain problems. It promotes healthy skin and improves the appetite in cases of debilitation. The FDA recently increased the RDA from 200 to 400mg daily, and since 1998 is used to fortify some cereals and grain products. Studies show that women who are at risk for getting pregnant should take extra folic acid rather than wait until after their pregnancy is suspected or confirmed.

## $ Biotin

Biotin is used in the body for synthesis of ascorbic acid. It is essential for the normal metabolism of fats and proteins. It maintains healthy skin and is especially good for the health of hair follicles. The best natural sources are nuts, fruits, brewer's yeast and unpolished rice. This vitamin will rejuvenate hair follicles when taken by mouth or rubbed directly on the skin in a cream base. It may even re-grow a few hairs that have gone into early retirement. Hair will stand up straighter and have a healthier sheen.

## $$ Choline

Found in lecithin, brewer's yeast, fish soybeans (tofu, tempeh, miso), peanuts, beef liver, egg yolk, wheat germ, cauliflower, cabbage. This B type vitamin is an antioxidant and membrane stabilizer It is used for transport and metabolism of fats and cholesterol in the liver. It may prevent cardiovascular disease and detoxifies the liver, and helps for better transmission of nerve impulses. It prevents and treats memory loss and diseases of the nervous system, and can influence mood and depression (manic depressive), as well as strengthen capillary walls, accelerate blood flow, thereby lowering blood pressure. Also, used in aiding the treatment of gallstones.

Deficiency symptoms could cause high blood pressure, bleeding stomach ulcers, heart trouble, blocking of the tubes and hemorrhaging of the kidneys, hardening of the arteries, atherosclerosis, headaches, dizziness, ear noises, palpitations and constipation. Choline seems to work better when taken with Biotin.

## $$$$ Vitamin $CoQ_{10}$ (Ubiquinal)

Dr. Carl Fokers, considered the Linus Pauling of $CoQ_{10}$. has repeatedly requested that this substance needs to be elevated to the status of a vitamin. There have been solid scientific studies on the mechanism and actions of $CoQ_{10}$ since the early 1970s. The body makes some $CoQ_{10}$ for basic function but not enough, and this is particularly true during times of mental and physical stress. It acts as a premiere antioxidant and has no negative side effects. But it is expensive, as vitamins go.

An Italian study of 2,664 patients with heart failure - hearts that weren't pumping strong enough to keep up with bodily demands — showed that those given an average of 100mg showed a marked improvement compared with patients not taking it. Langsjoen published a study on Coenzyme $CoQ_{10}$ for dilated cardiomyopathy, which is a boggy heart unable to pump hard enough.

Interest in this chemical was stimulated by the discovery, in 1961, that blood levels of $CoQ_{10}$ correlate quite well with cancer and the stage of the cancer. Breast cancer, for instance, is associated with a decrease in the blood levels of $CoQ_{10}$. In cancers with a bad prognosis, there is a dramatic decrease in $CoQ_{10}$ levels. It works to aid the body in trying to heal itself. Hence, the slower progression of cancer and perhaps an alternative or adjunct to radiation and chemotherapy. It stimulates the immune system and aids the body to heal itself. In some poorly controlled studies, it was shown to have cured cancer. The dose is 60mg a day to prevent cancer and heart disease and up to 300mg a day. Coenzyme $CoQ_{10}$ is absorbed better in oils and should be taken in peanut butter. But it comes in a maple-flavored chewable wafer with Vitamin E in a 200mg size that many of my patients take with their morning coffee. Q-Gel, a more expensive but better absorbed preparation, has come on the market, and one third of the dosage works well.

Now that $CoQ_{10}$ is available, studies have shown low levels of it in overactive thyroids, either naturally induced or because of too much thyroid medicine. Congestive heart failure also depletes $CoQ_{10}$. The biggest offenders, though, may be the "statin" drugs used by doctors to fight cholesterol. There are six on the market now and more will be introduced in the future. They are (generically with brand name in parenthesis) Lovastatin (Mevacor™), Provastatin (Pravachol™), Simvastin (Zocor™), Cerivastatin (Baycol™), Fluvostatin (Lescol™) and Atorvastatin (Lipitor™). These drugs can cause diffuse muscle aches, weakness and sometimes upset stomach. $CoQ_{10}$ can alleviate these symptoms and give only the benefits of these cholesterol-lowering drugs. The statins can cause other problems perhaps not related to $CoQ_{10}$ deficiency such as hepatitis, muscle inflammation and rash. If any of these show up, the drug should be stopped immediately and the prescribing doctor should be consulted.

Another concern about a low $CoQ_{10}$ is a less efficient immune system with all that entails including infection, cancer, aging. In a recent study dubbed CARE (Coronary and Recurrent Events) in which Pravachol was used, there was a marked reduction of heart attacks and strokes but a higher incidence of breast cancer in women.

## $ Bioflavonoids

The bioflavonoids (flavonoids, isoflavones) are polyphenolic antioxidants. It is sometimes referred to as vitamin P and found in fruits and vegetables. Major sources are tea, onions, apples, yams, cucumbers, citrus fruits and berries. Although there are various types such as Kaemoferol, Myricetin, Apigenen, Luetolin, Resveratol and proanthycyanidin, the most popular is Quercetin. Proanthycanidin is distributed in the United States under the name Adoxynol™. Dr. David White, a researcher at the University of Nottingham in England, says it is 50 times more powerful than Vitamin E.

Without flavonoids, Vitamin C is mostly oxidized and less useful. The flavonoids protect the integrity of the capillary wall, reduce blood clots and inhibit the oxidation of bad cholesterol to protect the cholesterol from becoming part of the plaque in the artery. It also reduces the body's ability to absorb cholesterol from food, according to Dr. T. Chisaka at the Kyoto Pharmaceutical University in Japan.

Dr. Michael Herzog was heading a study of more than 12,000 elderly men conducted by the public health divisions of seven European countries. The study was showing that a high intake of flavonoids resulted in a 50 percent less risk of having heart problems compared to those with a low intake.

In a study published in *Lancet* (342:1007 1993) in 805 males aged 65 to 64, there was an inverse relationship between the amount of flavonoids ingested over the previous five years by a cross-check dietary history and coronary artery disease. In addition, flavonoids have been shown to be anti-inflammatory and to decrease the incidence of viral infections.

## $ Inositol

Found in lecithin, organ meats, wheat germ, whole grains, brewer's yeast, blackstrap molasses, peanuts, citrus fruit. Used with choline it helps to metabolize fats and cholesterol in the arteries and liver. It helps to promote the body's production of lecithin in the growth and cell survival of bone marrow, eye membranes and intestines. Used with vitamin E it may help nerve damage in certain forms of muscular dystrophy. In certain cases it may prevent thinning hair and baldness. Inositol assists with brain cell nutrition and when used with choline it may help with menstrual problems. It may maintain hair growth and can make graying hair darken.

There are no deficiencies officially recognized, however, deficiency may cause constipation, eczema, abnormalities of the eyes, hair loss and high cholesterol.

## $$ PABA

Found in liver, brewer's yeast, wheat germ, molasses, eggs, organ meats, yogurt, green leafy vegetables. PABA stimulates intestinal bacteria, which aids in production of pantothenic acid. It is a coenzyme in making blood cells and metabolizing protein and important for skin health, hair pigmentation and health of intestines. It may also help with vitiligo, restore hair from graying and is used for many skin conditions. It protects against ozone toxicity.

Similar to symptoms caused by a folic acid or pantothenic acid deficiency; also vitiligo, fatigue, irritability, depression, nervousness, headache, constipation and other digestive disorders.

## Vitamin T

Known as the "sesame seed factor," vitamin T is found in sesame seeds and egg yolks. We do not yet know exactly what this substance is, but it is thought to be helpful in preventing anemia and the hemolysis of red blood cells. Halavah, a high-protein food made from sesame seeds, helped keep the armies marching in the time of Alexander the Great.

## Vitamin U

As with vitamin T, not much is known about vitamin U either. It is found in raw cabbage, has no known toxicity, and may be helpful in healing ulcers of the skin and intestinal tract. The active nutrient is probably allantoin, which has tissue-healing power, and is found in herbs such as comfrey root, which is know to help heal and soothe the gastrointestinal mucosa. Cabbage, commonly consumed in long living groups such as the Hunzas, has been thought to be a very important enzyme food.

## Multivitamins

Could you get all the necessary vitamins (and supplements) in one pill? That was the question I asked myself before asking a pharmacist to see if he could do it for me. He worked on it and then reported that the pill was as big as a golf ball. There are products on the market that come close but they are three to fifteen pills a day. What we understand is best for you this year will change with future research. I recommend a nutritionist, a naturopathic doctor or an experienced nutritional medical doctor to periodically review your vitamin protocol. Recently I went to a four capsule product, Juice Plus™. This may not have all the wonderful micronutrients in the world, but in double blind studies helps as much as taking a golfball size or a handful of pills.

## II. MINERALS

### $ Boron

Found in fresh fruits and vegetables, Boron helps retain calcium in bones and prevents calcium and magnesium loss through the urine. It also helps bone mineralization and prevents osteoporosis. In post-menopausal women it increases estrogen naturally. Deficiency symptoms have not been officially recognized. The optimal Daily Amount is 1-3mg daily combined with calcium, magnesium. No RDA has been established.

### $ Calcium

Found in milk, egg yolk, fish or sardines (eaten with bones), yogurt, soybeans, green leafy vegetables (such as turnip greens, mustard greens, broccoli and kale), roots, tubers, seeds, soups and stews made from bones, blackstrap molasses, almonds, figs and beans. Recent literature suggests calcium from milk sources may actually cause osteoporosis (see page 290). Calcium maintains acid-alkaline balance in the body and normalizes contraction and relaxation of the heart muscles. Taken for strong bones and teeth therefore protecting against osteoporosis, rickets and osteomalacia. It helps to lower high blood pressure, lowers cholesterol and aids in preventing cardiovascular disease. Try it with vitamin C for relief of backaches, menstrual cramps and to sleep more soundly (a natural tranquilizer). It can help prevent cancer, especially colorectal cancer.

The deficiency symptoms are nervous spasms, facial twitching, weak feeling muscles, cramps, rickets, slow growth in children, osteoporosis (porous and brittle bones), osteomalacia (bone-softening disease), heart palpitations and slow pulse rate, height reduction, colon cancer.

The optimal Daily Amount is1,000-1,500mg with half to equal parts of magnesium. Some researchers say menopausal women need 1,500mg, with added boron and magnesium. RDA is 1,000mg daily for adults, 1,200mg during pregnancy and lactation, 1,200mg for males and females from age 11 to 24.

### $ Chloride

Found in salt (sodium chloride) and salt substitute (potassium chloride), we seldom need supplementation. Chloride stimulates production of hydrochloric acid for digestion and maintains fluid and electrolyte balance. Chloride has also been shown to assist liver function.

The deficiency symptoms include impaired digestion, loss of hair and teeth, rare as the body usually produces enough. The optimal daily amount has not been established. Do not confuse chlorine, an active form of chloride, used in American water systems, which is indeed dangerous.

### $ Chromium

Found in brewer's yeast, blackstrap molasses, black pepper, meat (especially liver), whole wheat bread and cereals, beets and mushrooms. Chromium helps stabilize blood sugar levels, therefore being effective against diabetes and hypogly-cemia. It aids in lowering cholesterol and increases level of high-density lipoproteins (HDLs) in humans (shown protective against cardiovascular disease). Chromium can increase lean muscle tissue while decreasing body fat. Deficiency symptoms include slowed growth, shortened life span, raised cholesterol levels, an array of symptoms related to low and high blood sugar such as diabetes and low blood sugar. The optimal daily amount is 200-400mcg of GTF (glucose tolerance factor) taken with other minerals. Chromium polynicotinate (chelated), which is considered better than chromium picolinate (chelated to picolinic acid) are natural forms. RDA has not been established. The National Research Council tentatively recommends 500-2300 mcg daily to be effective and serves to improve blood sugar in diabetics.

### $ Copper

Found in nuts, organ meats, seafood, mushrooms and legumes. Accompanied by iron and protein it is able to synthesize hemoglobin (red blood cells). It forms melanin (pigment in skin and hair) and helps to make connective tissues such as collagen and elastin. Copper has the ability to assist in lowering cholesterol, improves the immune system and maintain cellular structure. It may help as an anti-inflammatory against arthritis.

Deficiency symptoms include a mild anemia, loss of hair, loss of taste, general weakness, impaired respiration, brittle bones, chronic or recurrent diarrhea, premature greying of hair, low white blood cell count which leads to reduced resistance to infection, retarded growth, water retention, nervous irritability, high cholesterol, abnormal ECG patterns, development of ischemic heart disease, birth defects, miscarriage and neural tube defects. Antacid use creates copper deficiency. Very high amounts cause mood swings and depression. Extra amount of copper come from cookware, hair sprays, deodorants, and copper water pipes. Excess amounts cause insomnia, painful joints, and mental and physical fatigue.

Optimal Daily Amount: 2-3mg taken with zinc at a 10:1 or 15:1 ratio (zinc:copper). RDA is 2mg.

## $ Fluoride

Found added to drinking water. Fluoride is thought to be necessary for formation of strong bones and teeth and may protect against osteoporosis. Too much may cause fatigue, muscle pain and even cancer and mottled teeth. There are no deficiency states and hence no optimal daily amount. Do not take additional fluoride. It is found in various toothpastes and mouthwashes. Because of the problems with fluoride producing the above symptoms (fluoridosis) many health care worker's lobbies oppose adding it to drinking water. In high doses of which a prescription is needed, it is used to improve is one mineral density. Twenty-five mg of a slow-acting form three times a day is recommended.

## $$ Germanium

Germanium is a trace mineral occurring naturally in very small amounts in the soil and in certain foods and herbs, such as shiitake mushrooms, ginseng root, garlic, shelf fungus, and aloe vera. It has been used for its semiconductor properties in making computer chips. But, in humans the organic form has a variety of healthy giving effects. The inorganic form has very little mammalian form of Ge-132, or Ge-Oxy 132 has varying immunological actions, such as stimulating interferon production, stimulating macrophage and NK (natural killer) lymphocyte activity, and enhancing cell-mediated immunity. There is some suggestion that Ge-132 helps in pain relief; particularly dramatic relief has occurred in some cases of severe cancer pain. In both sick and normal humans, Ge-132 is virtually nontoxic. Germanium is currently considered a food supplement and is available in health food stores. Make sure that it is in this organo-germanium sesquioxide form. Amounts in supplements range from 25-150 mg. or are available as pure powder. Suggested dosages for treatment range from 50-100 mg. daily, and up to 3-6 grams daily. Allergies have also been reduced by the use of this nutrient, particularly those allergies that arise to foods.

## $ Hydrochloric Acid (HCl)

As mentioned earlier in the book, Hydrochloric acid is greatly reduced in 30% of individuals older than 60 years of age. The parietal cells of the stomach produce HCl and secrete it primarily in response to ingested protein or fat. Decreased HCl production may lead to poor digestion, with symptoms such as gas, bloating, and discomfort after rich meals. Some symptoms may actually mimic an ulcer and folks erroneously take ulcer medicine. An HCl supplement may improve digestion of meals containing protein and/or fat, though not for foods such as rice and vegetables, which are largely carbohydrate and thus need less HCl for digestion. Hydrochloric acid is available primarily as betaine hydrochloride. When a 5-10 grain (1 grain = 64 mg.) tablet is taken during a meal, it should help proteins break down into peptide and amino acids and fats into triglycerides. I ask my patients to increase their number of pills even up to five at a time if a lower number of pills do not work. Betaine may be used alone, in supplements, or along with pepsin or other digestive agents. A Heidelberg capsule, gastric pH test (which directly measures stomach acid) can be done to verify a low or high acidity; then a supplement can be administered to see what effect it has on stomach pH. One reason that stress can cause more rapid aging is that it diminishes HCl production and weakens digestion. Low HCl production is associated with many problems, to include iron deficiency anemia, B12 deficiency, osteoporosis decrease mineral absorption. With low stomach aid levels, there can be an increase in bacteria, yeasts, and parasites growing in the intestines. HCl is a stimulus to pancreatic secretions, containing the majority of enzymes that actively break down foods.

## $ Iodine (Iodide)

Found in seaweed (especially kelp), seafood, iodized salt and sea salt, eggs, garlic, turnip greens, watercress. Iodine stimulates the thyroid gland to produce thyroxin. It protects against toxic effects from radioactive material. It is needed in over a hundred enzyme systems such as energy production, nerve function and hair and skin growth. It is able to stimulate conversion of body fat to energy, regulating basal metabolic rate. Finally, iodine has the ability to relieve pain and soreness associated with fibrocystic breast disease and can loosen clogged mucous in breathing tubes, and is used in a saturated solution for this.

Deficiency does occur and causes goiter (characterized by enlarged thyroid gland which may thicken the neck, restrict breathing), hypothyroidism (low thyroid), physical and mental sluggishness, poor circulation and low vitality, dry hair and skin, cold hands and feet, obesity, cretinism (physical and mental retardation in children born to mothers deficient in iodine), and hearing loss.

The optimal daily amount is 150-300mcg. Liquid iodine for medicinal uses (as an antiseptic for wounds) should NOT be used orally. With the advent of making iodize salt available in this country, iodide deficiency disorder are unheard of in the industrialized world, but we could see it in the future if a person goes on a strict, reduced sodium diet.

## $ Iron

Found in liver, heart, kidney, lean meats, shellfish, dried beans, fruit, nuts, green, leafy vegetables, whole grains, blackstrap molasses. Iron is the essential mineral in hemoglobin and myoglobin (red pigment in muscles). It can cure and prevent iron-deficiency anemia and stimulates immunity. Iron is needed in muscular and athletic performance and as an aid in preventing fatigue.

Deficiency is anemia (pallor, weakness, persistent fatigue, labored breathing on exertion, headaches, palpitation), young children suffer diminished coordination, decrease attention span and memory, older children have poor learning, reading and problem-solving skills, depressed immune system with decreased ability to produce white blood cells to fight off infection, concave or spoon-like fingernails and toenails.

The optimal daily amount (RDA) is 10mg for men, 18mg for women. As a supplement, do not use inorganic iron (ferrous sulfate) with vitamin E. Organic iron, found as ferrous fumarate, ferrous citrate or ferrous gluconate. Men and non-menstruating women should not take extra iron products in that it causes premature atherosclerosis since it is an oxidant.

## Lithium

Lithium is usually found in nature not as a metal but as a salt. *Lithos*, the Greek word for "stone," since the lithium crystals are beautiful and very hard rocks. Aside from hydrogen, lithium is the lightest element in use. It is used in medical treatment of manic-depressive disorders and as a mood stabilizer, commonly as lithium carbonate. Some natural mineral waters are high in lithium, as is the spirits, and soothe the digestion. Sugar cane and seaweed have been shown to contain lithium. It is thought to stabilize serotonin transmission in the nervous system; it influences sodium transport; and it may even increase lymphocytic (white blood cell) proliferation and depress the suppressor cell activity, thus strengthening the immune system.

Lithium toxicity is a very real possibility when it is used as a medicine. It is given in therapeutic doses only by prescription, with blood levels followed closely. Symptoms of lithium toxicity include nausea, vomiting, diarrhea, thirst, increased urination, tremors, drowsiness, confusion, delirium, and muscle weakness. There is no specific RDA for lithium. A therapeutic intake can vary from 300-1,500 mg. daily, though usually 300 mg. of lithium carbonate.

## $ Magnesium (Mg)

In a recent study, 75% of Americans were found to be deficient in magnesium. This is not your fault, but with modern agriculture, our soil has been depleted of his important mineral. Drugs such as diuretics, cortisone and aminophylline also lower our body's magnesium content. Magnesium also improves one's insulin and cholesterol metabolism and hence, will lower blood sugar and cholesterol. It is now thought to be as important as calcium to prevent osteoporosis. It has also successfully been used to treat PMS, mitral valve polapse, kidney stones, hypertension and migraine headaches. Deficiency syndromes include heart problems, apathy, depression, kidney stones, disorientation, muscle weakness and spasms, poor memory, irritability, tremors, and even seizures. Mg functions as a catalyst in over 1000 of our enzyme systems.

Although magnesium can be found in foods to include chard (150 mg magnesium/cup), pinto beans (95 mg magnesium/cup), avocados (70 mg each) and oatmeal (54 mg/cup), I recommend supplements. There are many products on the market such as Slo-Mag, Mag-L, K-Mag, Magnate and Magtab SR. This can be purchased in health food stores or inexpensively from the hardware store in the form of Epsom Salts. This is magnesium sulfate and $1/4^{th}$ teaspoon two or three times a day can supply you with the correct amount of magnesium. However, people occasionally do get a little diarrhea with this. Epsom Salt has been used in the past as a laxative. Periodically, the clinician should do a magnesium level to make sure the level is good without excess. However, in general, magnesium is a very safe mineral. There is some controversy over the analysis if the laboratory should obtain a serum, a red blood cell, or a white blood cell magnesium level. Although much more expensive, the white blood cell magnesium reflects the true body amount. The RDA is 400 mg daily and our diet supplies only half of that. Taken before bedtime gives a better night's sleep.

## $ Manganese

Manganese is found in whole grains, wheat germ, bran, peas, nuts, leafy green vegetables, beets, egg yolks, bananas, liver, organ meats, milk. It is required for vital enzyme reaction and proper bone development as well as synthesis of mucopoly-saccharides. It is helpful with osteoarthritis and is required for many enzyme reactions. The normal functioning of the pancreas needs manganese, as does carbohydrate metabolism. It plays an important part in the formation of thyroxin, a hormone secreted by the thyroid gland. It may also improve memory and reduce nervous irritability.

Deficiency symptoms include weight loss, dermatitis, nausea, slow growth and color changes of hair, low cholesterol, disturbances in fat metabolism and glucose tolerance, deficiency suspected in diabetes, deficiency during pregnancy may be a factor in epilepsy in the offspring, myasthenia gravis (severe loss of muscle strength). Too much will cause hypertension and irreversable movement disorders. Optimal Daily Amount: 5-10mg in combination with other minerals. No RDA has been established.

## $ Molybdenum

Molybdenum is found in organ meats (liver, kidney), milk, dairy products, legumes, whole grains, leafy green vegetables. This mineral is required for the activity of several enzymes in the body, a vital part of the enzyme responsible for iron utilization. It helps prevent anemia and detoxifies potentially hazardous substances with which one may come in contact. It can be an antioxidant and protects teeth from cavities. Finally it aids in carbohydrate and fat metabolism.

Deficiency symptoms include possible esophageal cancer in those who eat plants from molybdenum deficient soil. Optimal Daily Amount: Optimal intake is still uncertain; 50-200mcg (not mg). No RDA has been established.

## $ Phosphorous

This is found in high-protein foods such as meat, fish, poultry, eggs, milk, cheese, nuts, legumes, bone meal; many processed foods and soft drinks preserved with phosphates adversely affect the body's calcium phosphorous balance. Phosphorous is essential for bone mineralization, for normal bone and tooth structure. It may help with muscular fatigue and is involved in cellular activity. It has been shown to be important for heart regularity and needed for the transference of nerve impulses. Also aids in growth and body repair.

Deficiency symptoms include muscle weakness (to the point of respiratory arrest), anemia, increased susceptibility to infection. The typical diet usually makes a phosphorous deficiency rare in the United States, those with kidney failure or drink large quantities of pop can have too much. Alcoholics, diarheal diseases, and those taking antacids may be deficient. No supplementation needed as the diet should supply sufficient amounts. RDA is 800-1,200mg for adults.

## $ Potassium (K)

It is found in bananas, apricots, lettuce, broccoli, potatoes, fresh fruits and fruit juices, sunflower seeds, unsalted peanuts, nuts, squash, wheat germ, brewers yeast, desiccated liver, fish, bone meal, watercress, blackstrap molasses, and dried fruits. Potassium helps balance fluid with sodium inside the cells and used by the body for proper muscle and heart contraction. It helps red blood cells in carrying oxygen and eliminate water waste through kidneys. It is use in carbohydrate metabolism and energy storage in the muscles and liver. It reduces high blood pressure, allergies, colic in babies and is important for those using diuretics. Finally, it keeps the heart in rhythm.

Deficiency symptoms include general weakness of muscles, mental confusion, muscle cramping, poor reflexes, nervous system disruption, soft, flabby muscles, constipation, acne in young people, dry skin in adults. Severe deficiency or excess leads to cardiac arrest. The optimal daily amount is 2,000-4,000mg. Generally one gets enough from foods. Athletes generally require more (3,000-6,000mg) because of heavy perspiration. The maximum potency allowed by the government in supplement form is 99mg. Discuss higher potencies with a physician. RDA is 2,000-2,500mg. Expect the doctor to talk in milliequivalents (meq).

## $ Selenium

This is found in organ meats, tuna, seafood, brewer's yeast, fresh garlic, mushrooms, wheat germ and some whole grains. Selenium is necessary for the body's growth and protein synthesis. It helps to increase effectiveness of vitamin E. An antioxidant for the cells to protect against oxygen exposure, it also protects against toxic pollutants for sexual reproduction. Selenium may reduce risk of cancer and help against abnormal heart rhythm. It has been shown to alleviate hot flashes and some menopausal symptoms as well as reduce free-radical damage that causes aging.

Deficiency symptoms include dandruff, damaging effects of ozone in the lungs, decreased growth, infant deaths associated with selenium and/or vitamin E deficiency, and increased risk of cancer and heart disease. The Optimal Daily Amount is 100-200 ug in high selenium areas and 200-400 ug in low selenium areas. The Food and Nutrition Board states that overt selenium toxicity may occur in humans ingesting 3,000 ug a day. No RDA has been established. Up to 2 grams a day have been used in a series of cancer patients without apparent toxicity. I have used 600 ug of selenium for years in patients who have had disordered heart rhythm for years without apparent ill effects.

## $ Silver (See page 208)

## $ Silicon (Silica)

This is found in flaxseed, steel cut oats, almonds, peanuts, sunflower seeds, onions, alfalfa, fresh fruit, brewer's yeast and dietary fiber. Silicon can help build connective tissue. Most people take silica as a form of silicon, to help with hair, skin and nails.

Deficiency symptoms are aging of skin (wrinkles), thinning or loss of hair, poor bone development, soft or brittle nails. Optimal Daily Amount: No dietary recommendations. Adequate amounts are found in the diet. No RDA has been established.

## $ Sodium (Sodium Chloride, NaCl, Salt)

Found in sea salt, most foods from animal sources, shellfish, meat poultry, milk, cheese, kelp, powdered seaweed, most processed foods. Sodium works with potassium to maintain proper fluid balance between cells. Used for nerve stimulation for muscle contraction and helps in keeping calcium and other minerals soluble in the blood. Stimulates the adrenal glands and helps weak muscles. High sodium may accounts for high blood pressure and osteoporosis. Finally, sodium aids in preventing heat prostration or sunstroke. Deficiency is rare since most foods contain sodium, however, symptoms include headaches, excessive sweating, heat exhaustion, respiratory failure, muscular cramps, weakness, collapsed blood vessels, stomach and intestinal gas, chronic diarrhea, weight loss, kidney failure, and a tendency for infections. A gram of sodium chloride has been suggested for each kilogram of water ingested. RDA is 200-600mg. In our modern society, we take too much of this mineral into our bodies. Home water softeners prepared foods and the salt shakers are the worst offenders. If we did not have any salt consumption there would be no hypertension.

## $ Sulfur

This is found in protein foods, especially eggs, lean beef, fish, onions, kale, soybeans, dried beans. Sulfur is in every cell of the body, helping the nerves and muscles function properly, and normalizing glandular secretions. It is necessary for healthy hair, skin and nails. It also helps maintain oxygen balance necessary for brain function. The homeopathic remedy of sulfur helps with rashes and itching and other skin conditions. Deficiency symptoms are rare but may be excessive sweating, chronic diarrhea, nausea, respiratory failure, heat exhaustion, muscular weakness and mental apathy. A diet sufficient in protein should be adequate in sulfur. No RDA has been established. MSM (see page 236) is an excellent source of extra sulfur taking in 500 to 1,000 mg a day supplement.

## $ Vanadium

This is found in fish, black pepper and dill seed, the richest sources; middle range is whole grains, meats and dairy products. Research showed that it improved glucose tolerance and improved efficiency in insulin in diabetics. Deficiency symptoms are little known at this time, but high blood pressure and hardening of the arteries have been suggested.

No RDA has been established, but 10 to 50 mg a day for diabetes of Vanadium sulfate are recommended.

## $ Zinc

This is found in fresh oysters (which are really dangerous to eat), herring, wheat germ, pumpkin seeds, milk, steamed crab, lobster, chicken, pork chops, turkey, lean ground beef, liver, eggs. Zinc helps promote wound healing and helps improve acne. It affects impotence in men and aids in increasing sperm count. It helps for prostate enlargement problems. Use for combating colds and flu to increase immunity, it may help with some forms of cancer and is helpful for macular degeneration along with antioxidants (see page 118).

Deficiency symptoms are fingernails with white spots or bands or an opaquely white appearance, loss of taste, smell and appetite, delayed sexual development in adolescence, underdeveloped penis and less full beard and underarm hair in boys, irregular menstrual cycle in girls, infertility and impaired sexual function in adults, poor wound healing, loss of hair, increased susceptibility to infection, reduced salivation, skin lesions, stretch marks, reduced absorption of nutrients, impaired development of bones, muscles and nervous system, deformed offspring and dwarfism. Given to a teenager, it might make the youngster taller. Optimal Daily Amount: 30-50mg (take with copper, a zinc:copper ratio of 10:1). RDA is 15mg. I frequently prescribe 200-250 mg a day).

## III. HERBAL PREPARATIONS
### Algae

Algae are green, or "blue-green," freshwater, one-celled organisms grown, dried, and safely used by our bodies. Chlorella, spirulina, and blue-green manna are three of the main products produced from algae. All of these blue-green algae, or plankton products, have been used as "high protein" nutrients that contain all the amino acids. They are considered a tonic and/or rejuvenator of the body and are used commonly during weight-loss programs or fasting. Decreased appetite, weight loss, and improved energy levels, especially mental are also claimed. Besides the high protein and low fat levels of these algae, they contain substantial amounts of vitamins and minerals and plant chlorophyll; spirulina was recently measured as rich in GLA, or gamma-linolenic acid, the oil found in the evening primrose plant.

## $ Aloe Vera

Aloe vera, which has been used by the South American Indians for the last two millenniums, is still an effective way to treat skin disorders. An enzyme that inactivates the healing products (acemannon) once the leaf is cut is the reason for the leaf to be used fresh. Therefore, previously prepared products may be ineffective. I recommend using the live aloe vera plant such as the ancients did. One could pull off a leaf, and with scissors cut off a portion from the bottom (as much of the leaf as is needed to cover the lesion). The leaf is pulled apart and "pasted" on the skin much like a band-aid. The rest of the leaf is put in water to keep the remainder of the leaf fresh and rejuvenated for the next time it is used. This step is repeated once or twice a day until the entire leaf is gone. If needed, pull off another leaf. Additionally, if eaten raw, aloe vera may heal peptic ulcers and other digestive disorders, as well as help the body fight off illness and prevent cancer. It also works as a mild laxative. This natural product contains germanium, which my be another reason for its healing benefits.

The aloe plant is easily cultivated outdoors and in the early fall there are many daughter plants. These are brought in to be used until next spring brings out new leaves on your winter dormant plant. If you choose, one can buy long leaf aloe vera at a Chinese grocery or a health food store. You can ingest the aloe plant for months for chronic bowel, immune and degenerative disorders.

### Taking Aloe Vera Orally
1. Obtain an 18 to 24-inch leaf of aloe vera leaf or several smaller home grown leaves.

2. Cut one inch long piece off the tip of the leaf.
3. Cover the cut surface of the leaf with a piece of cellophane and put it in the refrigerator.
4. Fillet the cut piece (first cut off the edges with spine, then peel the skin).
5. Cut the piece of peeled aloe into three parts (it looks like colorless jello).
6. Put two of the three pieces of peeled aloe in a zip-lock bag and refrigerate.
7. Cut the third piece into six parts. Take each piece separately, taking a large swallow of water with each piece of aloe. Chewing the aloe piece is neither necessary nor desirable due to its taste.
8. Take the two refrigerated pieces at lunch and dinner times, or other convenient times.

NOTE: The first piece of aloe should be about one-half the size of sugar cube so that gagging, if it occurs, is not too uncomfortable. Once you get used to it, you may take aloe in suitably larger pieces.

## $$ Ashwagandha

Ashwagandha, a rich continental Indian or Ayurvedic herb, has been shown to boost the body's immune and resistance to disease, which, in effect, slows the aging process. It also seems to improve nervous system function; practitioners use it to treat patients who are physically or mentally stressed. (It seems to work by regulating the release of cortisol, a hormone that we produce when we're under stress.) Ashwagandha is also used to help age-related memory problems, and it has been shown to improve libido in men. For people who have arthritis, ashwagandha contains a natural anti-inflammatory to help ease pain.

Some compounds in ashwagandha have been found to increase the ability of mice and rats to learn and retain memories. Withaferin A, a compound in ashwagandha, has been shown to fight tumors, viruses, bacteria, and fungal infections. Withaferin A also has antiarthritic and anti-inflammatory activity.

To help diminish some of the effects of aging, or for general strengthening purposes, take 250-500 mg of standardized ashwagandha extract in tablets morning and night.

## $$ Bacopa

Bacopa is an Ayurvedic herb that is a general antioxidant but specifically increases memory, especially verbal. The active chemical in the herb is bacoside A, which increases brain acetylcholine. Acetylcholine decreases have been implicated as the major mechanism as a cause of Alzheimer's disease. Bacopa neutralizes the neurotoxins produced by stressors, such as excess adrenaline that may be at the root of neurodegeneration. Also, this herb may prevent or retard Parkinson's disease in those predisposed to this. Most of all as an anti-aging agent it helps to increase novelty seeking behavior, which is an attribute of intelligence associated with increased mental pleasure and lifespan. In this respect, it decreases anxiety, mental fatigue, and attention deficit, promoting vigilance and task performance. It is available in health food stores for about $15.00 for a months supply of a capsule three times a day. It is safe and has no major side effects, except a rare mild allergic reaction.

## $$ Bilberry

The anthocyanosides in bilberries can improve circulation, protect fragile capillaries and delay vital chemical destruction in the eye; they have a positive effect on enzymes crucial to vision and the eye's ability to adapt to the dark. It may improve diabetes and heart disease. Although scientists don't know what components of the bilberry leaf are responsible for these effects, recent research has shown that taking a dried leaf extract will cause a drop in glucose (blood sugar) levels. The same research also showed that bilberry leaf can lower blood triglyceride levels, a heart disease risk factor.

The most popular products are extracts standardized to contain 15 to 25 percent of a chemical called anthocyanosides. Bilberry is also available as tinctures and concentrated drops. An average dose of an encapsulated extract standardized for 20 to 25 percent anthocyanosides is 60 to 120mg. The herb's short-term effect on vision is most noticeable within the first four hours of taking it; thus it can be useful if taken before a visually demanding task like driving all night or reading the entire Sunday paper.

Tests have shown bilberry to be completely nontoxic, even when taken in large doses for an extended period of time. In England the Bilberry fruit is eaten for almost the same effect. In the U.S., bluberries are almost as good as the bilberry. The bilberry is blue through and through and hence has more of the anthocyanoside than the blueberry that has it just under the "skin."

## $ Calendula

The plant contains several beneficial chemicals, including flavonoid, a gelatinous substance called mucilage, an essential oil and alcohols. While scientists are still determining which of these constituents does what, researchers in Japan last year isolated and identified alcohol constituents from calendula flowers that showed marked anti-inflammatory activity. Skin irritations, superficial wounds and insect bites and stings all respond well to calendula.

Calendula is sold in liquid forms (such as juice, concentrated drops and tinctures) and as an ingredient in herbal combination ointments, salves, lotions and creams. It is also used to make homeopathic calendula remedies and an essential oil, both of which are used topically to treat skin irritations, burns and scrapes. (An easy way to use the herb is to soak a gauze pad in calendula tincture and apply directly to the skin.)

Calendula has not been associated with toxicity or side effects.

## $ Cayenne

The medicine chemical in cayenne I capsaicin. Capsaicin appears to alter the action of the bodily compound (called "substance P") that transfers pain messages to the brain,

186

of pain and inflammation. Beyond this, a recent study found that cayenne has antimicrobial effects, meaning it could be used to fight infections. When taken orally, cayenne stimulates circulation, aids digestion and promotes sweating. (Because perspiration works to cool the body, cayenne is sometimes used to break a fever.)

Cayenne contains a compound called capsaicin, which is the active ingredient in many over-the-counter and prescription creams used to treat arthritis, shingles (herpes zoster), post-operative pain, cluster headaches, psoriasis and other skin conditions. Cayenne is the ingredient of hot peppers, either the fruit or a prepared product. (See "Fire in the Hole" page 91). Cayenne is also sold in capsules, concentrated drops and tinctures, which are taken orally. Popular products are standardized for 5 to 10 percent capsaicin. An average dose of an oral extract standardized for eight percent capsaicin is 100mg.

Cayenne is potent and can cause serious tissue irritation if used improperly. Be sure to wash your hands thoroughly after using capsaicin-containing creams; avoid any contact with eyes, mucous membranes, or open wounds. Excessive internal use can inflame the membranes that line the stomach and intestines and harm the kidneys. Follow label's directions carefully and don't exceed the recommended doses. One can easily make their own capsaicin from red or cayenne pepper.

## $$ Chamomile

German Chamomile, to be distinguished from Roman chamomile, can be used to help one relax and it's also a reliable remedy for skin irritation. It improves tissue regeneration, reduces inflammation and stimulates the immune-boosting activity of white blood cells, thanks to the action of chemical flavonoids. Apigenin, a flavonoid derived from chamomile, was found to have anti-anxiety and mild sedative effects. It is mildly anti-inflammatory due to its antiprostaglandin effect (a hormone-like substance that influences nerve conduction).

Chamomile comes as a dried whole herb (to be used as a

tea or bath infusion) and in packaged teas, tables, capsules, concentrated drops, tinctures and extracts. Follow dosage directions on labels.

Both oral and topical chamomile products are considered very nontoxic, gentle enough for use in children, or during pregnancy and lactation. An extremely remote concern is that people with an allergy to some other herb in the daisy family would also be allergic to chamomile. Chamomile-based skin creams should not come in contact with eyes.

## $$ Cranberry

Researchers studying cranberry's abilities to fight urinary tract infections at first suspected that the juice made urine more acidic, which made the urinary tract less hospitable to bacteria. However, recent studies indicate that the herb prevents bacteria from sticking to the lining of the urinary tract and does kill bacteria. Cranberry is rich in flavonoids, citric and other acids and vitamin C; exactly which compounds are most active in promoting good urinary tract health (and delivering cranberry's other health benefits) is still being determined.

Most tablets and capsules contain dried, unsweetened juice powder or concentrated extract. An average dose is 500 to 1,000mg per day. Unsweetened cranberry juice (available in some health foods stores) is the most potent cranberry drink, but many people find it difficult to get down; sweetened drinks are more palatable. "Cranberry juice drinks" typically contain 10 to 20 percent juice; "cranberry juice cocktails" typically have 25 to 35 percent real juice. Some observers have wondered whether these products were too diluted or sugar-laden to have any therapeutic effects but a number of recent studies have found that they can be quite beneficial. For instance, a 1994 study found that 10 ounces per day of commercially available cranberry juice cocktail was almost twice as effective as a placebo in reducing bacteria in urine. When buying the "juice drinks," one will have to drink roughly twice the amount, 20 ounces a day. Cranberry extract is available in capsules or tablets.

## $$ Echinacea

Echinacea (pronounced Eke-nay-shuh) is an extremely important herb used for enhancing the immune system. As such, it has been used for viral infections such as colds to AIDS, as well as the treatment of mild maladies of unknown cause, such as the chronic fatigue syndrome and/or fibromyalgia. The herb, which is a flower (Echinacea Purpurea) is sometimes referred to as a "Purple Kansas Cone Flower," grows the best out of the whole world in the state of Kansas. It ahs been used for over 500 years by the American Indians and in the last century has been used commonly in the Orient as well as in Europe. In the year 2000, over 10,000 pounds were exported to Europe. The plant (herb) is extremely safe and can be grown at home or obtained from the health food store without a prescription. It is available in pills, tea, powders, or in drops. Unlike an antibiotic or an anti-viral drug (Tamaflu, Relenza), this drug is used more as a preventative and helps the body's own forces to ward off disease. A cousin of Echinacea is Goldenseal. It seems to have a true anti-viral effect. Many people take both together. They are available both in a single capsule. One three times a day to prevent or treat a mild problem is recommended and twice that much whn very ill. There is no interference with these botanicals and any other medication.

## $ Elderberry

Most commonly used to treat the runny nose and sore throat of the common cold and to help to reduce the fever, muscle pain and other symptoms of the flu. Elderberry induces sweating and stimulates circulation; it also has slight laxative and cough-suppressant effects. The berries are rich in vitamin C, flavonoids such as anthocyanins, substances called tannins, and other phyto-nutrients. Certain compounds may help counter the effects of some strains of influenza by binding to the virus and preventing it from attacking cells. Recently, scientists tested a standardized extract of the berry, Sambucol (see page 206), found that it caused a complete cure or at least a significant improvement in symptoms of the flu within two to three days.) The flowers contain flavonoids, an essential oil, mucilage, tannins and other compounds, whose main effects appear to be reducing fever and promoting sweating.

Elderberry comes in tinctures, liquid extracts, lozenges, syrups, standardized extract capsules and throat sprays. Follow dosage directions on labels. Herbal products made from the leaves or bark of the elderberry tree should NOT be taken internally.

## $$$$ Ellagic Acid

Ellagic acid is a naturally occurring constituent in certain fruits and nuts especially with red raspberries and strawberries. It has been touted as an effective anti-mutagen (prevents birth defects) and inhibitor of cancer. It also promotes wound healing, reduces and reverses chemically induced liver fibrosis, and is a potent antioxidant. As an antioxidant, it might benefit a number of degenerative diseases. It also has anti-bacterial and anti-viral properties. The product is proprietary and one capsule is equivalent to eating, one cup of pureed raspberries. The usual dose is four to eight capsules per day in divided doses. Ellgic Red 4 is available from 21st Century (1-800-638-7462 or www.21stcn.com).

## Essiac

Essiac is a four herb remedy of burdock root (*Arctium appa*), the inner bark of slippery elm (*Ulmus fulva*), sheep's sorrel (*Rumex acetosella*), and Turkish rhubarb root (*Rheum palmatum*) usually made in a tea. The remedy was given to Rene Caisse, a Canadian nurse by an Ojibway Indian herbalist shortly before World War I. She subsequently treated hundreds of patients in the ensuing sixty years. Essiac is Caisse spelled backwards. Although originally thought of as a cure for cancer, it has had more than a modicum of success in treating peptic ulcers, lupus, thyroid disease, type 2 diabetes, and AIDS. The cancers that it seems to work best on are prostate, colon, breast, lung, and ovarian. The herbs do improve the immune system and as such may well be anti-aging. It is available form the Herbal Healer Academy, Inc., HC 32, Box 97-B, Mt. View, AR. 72560, phone 870-269-4177, costing $25.00 for enough herb to make 200 gallons taking 2 oz., three times a day. Additionally, one can buy the individual herbs separately at most health food stores. This product reputedly is extremely safe with only a rare allergic reaction.

### $ Evening Primrose

Known botanically as *Oenothera biennis*, oil of evening primrose (OEP) is used by women to help relieve breast pain and symptoms of the premenstrual syndrome (PMS). OEP is also believed by some to decrease the risk of other conditions, such as cardiovascular disease and rheumatoid arthritis. The effects of OEP are attributed to its high concentrations of the fatty acids cis-linoleic acid and cis-y-linolenic acid (GLA). Both are produced in the body in limited amounts.

Women with breast pain have reduced levels of GLA (most likely secondary to decreased conversion of cis-linoleic acid to GLA). Supplementation of 2.4 to 3.2 g/d of OEP (in divided doses) has been shown to decrease pain in 44% of women with cyclical breast pain and 27% of those with noncyclical breast pain. OEP must be taken for at least four months before its effects will be felt, because its onset is delayed. Women with PMS are also believed to have decreased conversion of cis-linoleic acid to GLA. The resulting reduction in GLA levels leads to deficient synthesis of prostaglandin E1, which is thought to aggravate PMS Symptoms. In one study, administration of 4 capsules of OEP (each containing 72% linoleic acid and 9% GLA) twice daily during the last 14 days of the menstrual cycle relieved PMS symptoms. However, conclusive results concerning the effectiveness of OEP for PMS are lacking, because other studies have shown no effect. It is good for HRT and tender breasts.

OEP is relatively free of side effects, although mild gastrointestinal irritation has been reported. OEP has no known drug interactions. Most studies evaluating the use of OEP have used products containing 72% cislinoleic acid and 9% GLA. Patients should use the brand of OEP that contains these amounts of fatty acids, and they should follow the manufacturer's guidelines for dosing.

## $ Feverfew

Feverfew's principal traditional use was to reduce fever but it also has a long history of treating headaches. It is also used to reduce the inflammation of arthritis and to relieve menstrual pain. Researchers have determined in a number of placebo-controlled human studies that feverfew can reduce the frequency and severity of migraines. The herb appears to inhibit some of the negative (and migraine-related) effects of certain chemicals that are produced by the body, including histamines and the brain chemical, serotonin. Scientists have traced feverfew's antimigraine action to chemicals known as lactone compounds (parthenolide in particular, although exactly how parthenolide works is still being determined).

Feverfew is sold dried and in capsules, concentrated drops, tinctures and extracts. The newest products are standardized for 0.1 to 0.2 percent of the chemical. parthenolide. An average daily dose is 125mg of feverfew (standardized for 0.2 percent parthenolide) or 250mcg parthenolide. Note: A number of studies done in the last 10 years indicate that several commercial feverfew products contained none of the active compound parthenolide in addition, parthenolide levels of the dried herb were found to fall during storage. These studies emphasized the importance of using high-quality standardized extracts of this herb for proper dosage and reliable effects.

## $ Garlic

Garlic has been an important part of life for centuries, across cultures and millennia. No other single food has had as many applications as this pungent plant. Studies show that garlic protects against infection and inflammation, lowers the risk of heart disease, hypertension and has anti-cancer and anti-aging effects. Garlic does not have to be eaten raw or fresh to be effective. The potent odor of garlic may not be necessary for its health benefits. Research show that aged, deodorized garlic extract sometimes works even better than fresh garlic without causing digestive disorders and "garlic breath" that may haunt the fresh garlic eater. Long before humans began keeping written records, garlic, found in the wild, was cultivated for human use. Though the exact geographic origin of garlic is not known, modern botanists think it came from Central Asia, some say Siberia. The plant, with its pungent flavored bulb, was transported West and East by migrating tribes, becoming native to Mediterranean regions of Europe, Asia and Africa as well as China and other countries in the far East. The history of garlic stretches far back, to a time when people who foraged in the fields for food and healing herbs came across garlic and cultivated it for their use. Remnants of garlic have been found in cave dwellings that are over 10,000 years old. In India, Ayurvedic medicine recommends garlic to boost energy and treat colds and fatigue.

Garlic, *Allium sativum,* is a hardy perennial plant that belongs to the lily family, as do onions, leeks, shallots and chives. However, garlic contains a number of organosulfur substances with medicinal properties that are unique to it. Some Chinese eat about 20 grams of garlic a day, approximately 8 medium size cloves. In some European countries, most adults take a daily garlic supplement to promote health. In the United States the use of garlic preparations as supplements has been rapidly escalating in recent years, as is easily detected in crowd. The chemistry of garlic is complex, with over 100 different compounds that contribute to its effects. The most important and unique feature is its high content of organosulfur substances. Garlic contains at least four times more sulfur than other high sulfur vegetables-onion, broccoli, and cauliflower.

From a medicinal point of view, the most important organosulfur substance are water soluble S-allyl cysteine and other sulfur amino acids that are increased by aging garlic extract. Stable, odorless and safe, with high antioxidant activity, S-allyl cysteine easily gets into the circulatory system from the gut (highly bioavailable), with an absorption of close to 90%. S-allyl cysteine has been shown to slightly reduce blood cholesterol levels, protect cells from toxic chemicals, prevent cancer in laboratory animals and stop the growth of prostate cancer cells and breast cancer cells, in culture. Its high antioxidant activity provides it with the potential to fight oxidant-related damage that leads to heart disease, cancer and aging. Non-sulfur compounds in garlic and in the aged extract include proteins, carbohydrates (sugars, fructans, pectins), saponins, that are steroid substances recently shown to have antibacterial and antifungal actions, flavonoids, such as allixin, that are important antioxidants. Garlic contains low amounts of vitamins and minerals including selenium. The organosulfur compounds are mostly responsible for garlic's medicinal qualities, but their cooperative action with other components that are present in garlic enhances its health benefits. The odorific chemical is absorbed into the blood stream, metabolized and is excreted in the sweat and breath more unpleasant odor than the original herb.

Garlic comes in four forms, fresh garlic, garlic powder, garlic oil, and aged garlic extract (Kyolic™). Fresh garlic has a pungent lingering odor and a burning sensation due to the release of allicin, which is produce upon the first bite into the whole clove. Garlic powder is made by drying sliced garlic cloves. The powder contains some alliin and alliinase that produce allicin when mixed with water. Garlic powder provides oil soluble organosulfur compounds that provide health benefits. However, the amounts may vary widely with the manufacturer. It is best to use a standardized high-allicin garlic powder and take it with a fatty-meal or, ideally, with fish, flax or Perilla oil supplements for optimal assimilation. Steamed distilled crushed raw garlic is diluted with vegetable oils to make garlic oil. The processing in part reduces garlic's pungent odor, which is why garlic oil contains only a fraction of the original garlic oil soluble sulfides. It does not contain water soluble sulfur compounds and , because of high heat distillation, non volatile garlic nutrients are lost.

Produced from organically grown garlic by gentle alcohol extraction and aging, the extract lasts up to 20 months. No heating is applied. The aging process retains garlic nutrients, produces large amounts of water soluble S-allyl cysteine and S-allylmercaptocysteine and converts unstable substances such as allicin to stable compounds that are odorless and beneficial. These include some oil soluble and some water soluble organosulfur compounds. S-allyl cysteine and S-allyl mercaptocysteine are present in the aged extract at higher levels compared with fresh garlic. Standardized by levels of S-allyl cysteine, aged garlic extract provides a safe and stable product that has encouraged many researchers to favor this supplement in studying the health effects of garlic.

## $ Ginger

Zesty flavor notwithstanding, ginger is often used for its calming effects on a upset stomach. It is also used to treat nausea and motion sickness. In some people it also can help reduce a fever or lessen the symptoms of a cold and arthritis. Also, it is a very mild anticoagulant, potent antioxidant, and has a claim for being an energizer and antiaging. Ginger contains essential oils including gingerol and shogaol that are responsible for its medicine properties. Ginger comes in a variety of forms including candies, fresh, dried, tablets, capsules, tinctures, extracts, syrups and teas; follow dosage directions on labels. You can also buy ginger essential oil, which can be diffused into the air for inhalation or diluted in a vegetable oil for topical application (or massage). The fresh root can be used, but it is quite sharp. Ginger from the spice shelf is very handy and useful. Three to four shakes in ginger ale or club soda has worked for a number of my patients.

Ginger has a long history of being taken in relatively large doses (up to several grams) without causing any toxicity or side effects. Many pregnant women use it to help control morning sickness, but there have been no studies in which women have taken large doses of ginger during pregnancy. Do not ingest the essential oil and be sure to dilute it before applying to your skin. The fresh root is very spicy.

## $$ Gingko Biloba

According to the *Journal of American Medical Association*, October 22/29, 1997, Volume 278, November 16, a double blind study was performed at Albert Einstein College of Medicine in New York, which revealed that Ginkgo Biloba was safe and capable of stabilizing as well as improving the thinking and social functioning of patients with "mild memory loss." Unlike the prescription "ethical drugs," this is an herb that can be bought at pharmacies and health food stores. The herb itself is from the gingko tree, which is one of the oldest trees still in existence today, going back 280 million years!! This has been used for a millennium in Chinese medicine and for centuries in Europe, particularly Germany. It has recently been approved in that country for the treatment of dementia. For the last 8 years I have been working with this botanical and similar to the research, I find it does have a definite benefit in as many as 40% of people taking this. Even in people who do not have a dementing disease, it seems to increase the memory and actually improve the IQ. It may take several months for the herb to show an effect and most of the time the effect is a subtle improvement.

Ginkgo is a mild antioxidant and may be useful in asthma, coughs, and allergies. The active flavinoid compound is flavoglycoside. It is supplied in encapsulated extracts that should be standardized to 24% of the flavoglycoside. The capsules come in 40 to 60 mg size and four to six a day are recommended. Rarely nausea, headache, a dizziness can occur. Although it is said to potentiate the anticoagulate warfarin (coumadin). I have never had a problem with it in many of my patients who have taken both together. Certainly one should tell their physician if they are taking Ginkgo and should not vary the dose without telling him. I had a single patient, a pharmacist, who had a nonspecific bleeding disorder on Gingko.

## $$$$ Glucarate
## (non-herbal and should be in the supplement section)

Glucarate is a detoxifying phytonutrient. Calcium D-Glucarate, a non-toxic sugar compound found in certain fruits (cherries, grapefruits, grapes, and apricots) and cruciferous vegetables. It is a normal constituent in tissues and body fluids. A growing body of research in animal models indicates that dietary Calcium D-Glucarate helps protect the body against many toxic compounds. The primary mechanism of action appears to be the ability of oral Calcium D-Glucarate to increase net elimination of certain toxic compounds following glucuronidation. Uncontrolled cell transformations and other tissue damage can result from exposure to foreign chemicals. Glucuronidation results in the detoxication and excretion of fat-soluble toxins and steroid hormones including xenoestrogens. Glucuronidation products formed in the liver can be deconjugated by B-glucuronidase, an enzyme produced by intestinal bacteria. This prevents the freed compound to be reabsorbed back into the body and reduces toxicity and hormonal dysregulation. Glucarate is extremely safe and large doses are needed to make a therapeutic impact in some cases. For consultation of dose and purchase call Tyler Labs at 1-800-869-9705 or Nutraceutix at 1-800-548-3222.

## $ Goldenseal

Goldenseal (*Hydrastis canadensis*) root has been a panacea and cure-all used by many herbalists and a very popular herb to the Native Americans. Its active alkaloids, hydrastine and berberine, appear to have many body actions. This bitter, tonifying herb is used as an antibacterial and antiparasitic, especially for giardia and amoebic infections. Many people take goldenseal capsules at the first sign of a flu or other infection and claim good results, this goldenseal powder has been used as a douche, gargle, or as a bitter tonic taken orally to strengthen the mucous membranes of the gastrointestinal tract, and insuflated in the sinuses and eyes. Two goldenseal capsules can be opened stirred in a half cup of warm water and inhaled through the nose for sinus and other respiratory infections, as well as used as an enema. Goldenseal is also an antiseptic and detoxifier, possibly because of its liver-stimulating effect. It has mild laxative and vasoconstrictive actions, making it useful in the treatment of hemorrhoids, both applied externally and taken internally. Goldenseal has been used for skin problems such as acne or eczema, as a uterine tonic, and to stimulate glandular activity and strengthen the nervous system. Goldenseal may be helpful for many problems of the stomach and gastrointestinal tract, such as nausea, indigestion, infection, and constipation or diarrhea; here it can also reduce bacterial (H. pylori) or parasitic proliferation, increase gastrointestinal tone, and stimulate bile secretion and digestion.

For most of these situations, goldenseal can usually be taken orally in capsules or liquid (or 10-20 drops of an extract) twice daily for about two to three weeks. Remotely long continuous intake of this herb can cause possible liver dysfunction, although I have never seen a single case in forty years of medical practice.

### $$ Ginseng, Panax

Panax Ginseng stands out from the other four varieties on the market (see page 207). It is used for folks over the age of 40, especially those experiencing stress, tension, exhaustion, fatigue, or debility. Dried root as tea or in tablets: 1 g or two 500 mg tablets, Tincture 1/5: 1 teaspoon; Fluid extract 1/1: 20 drops; Standardized extract: 100mg extract standardized to 4 to 7% ginsenosides. Take three times a day for three months continuously, then one month on two months off. This regime can be used indefinitely. It is a stimulant, but not an excitant. Panax will decrease LDL cholesterol and triglycerides. This herb could elevate the digoxin level in the test tube, but not your body, so tell your allopathic physician that you are taking this preparation.

## $ Green Tea

Studies indicate that green tea may help protect against cancers of the lungs, skin, liver, pancreas and stomach; it also boosts cardiovascular health and may work as a weight-loss agent by increasing fat metabolism and regulating blood sugar and insulin levels. Green tea benefits the heart by lowering cholesterol levels and reducing the tendency of blood platelets to stick together. It contains numerous cancer-fighting polyphenol compounds, including the antioxidant flavonoid catechin. The evidence for green tea's potent antioxidant effects continues to accumulate. In a recent study researchers found that green tea compounds not only directly scavenge free radicals but also enhance the effectiveness of the body's natural antioxidant systems. Green tea extract may promote weight loss, according to an article in the *American Journal of Clinical Nutrition* (1999; 70:1040-1045). The catechin polyphenol, which works with other chemicals, increases levels of fat oxidation and thermogenesis (where the body burns fuel, such as fat, to create heat). This increase in energy expenditure is probably the mechanism causing weight loss.

You can buy encapsulated extracts standardized for chemicals called polyphenols. An average dose is 200mg of an extract standardized for 25 percent polyphenols. One can also buy the dried herb and make tea; it's available in various grades, from twiggy, inexpensive kikich to choice sencha. Drink up to four or five cups of green tea per day. The most worrisome chemical in green tea is caffeine, but occurs in small amounts (an average of 20 to 30mg per cup, if brewed for two to three minutes). This is much less caffeine than in coffee, however; an 8-ounce cup of coffee. Black tea may be just as good according to a study in the 1999Archives of Internal Medicine (159: 2170-2174). In another study Boston's Dr. Joe Vita showed that nitric oxide is released by black tea and dilates the coronary arteries. However, do not add milk in that it reduces the availability of the active flavinoid.

## $ Hawthorn

Hawthorn helps the heart because it tends to normalize blood pressure, prevent palpitations and arrhythmias and relieve angina. Studies have confirmed that the plant is a rich source of healthy chemical compounds, including procyanidins and the flavonoids rutin and vitexin, which have been shown to dilate blood vessels of the heart and thus improve blood flow. These cardiovascular effects result from taking the herb over a prolonged period. Researchers in Germany recently gave hawthorn extract to patients suffering from congestive heart failure and found the patients experienced fewer overall symptoms and showed improvements in stamina and a reduction in blood pressure and heart rate during exercise. Hawthorn is good for arthritis because it helps stabilize collagen, the protein found in joints that are destroyed by inflammatory diseases. It also has antioxidant effects.

Hawthorn is sold as dried berries, capsules and tinctures. Extracts are often standardized for one of two different chemical compounds: total flavonoids usually calculated as vitexin or procyanidins. An average dose is 200mg of an extract standardized for approximately 1.5 percent vitexin or 2.0 percent flavonoids. The herb is considered non-toxic, consumers should be warned, though, that if you do take a digitalis prescription, this could elevate your blood level and should be monitored closely by your physician. However, no cases of toxicity have yet been reported.

## $ Hops

Hops *(Humulus lupulus)*, with its delicate female stobiles so often used as a flavoring in addition to preventing osteoporosis, helps folks fall to sleep easier. Moreover, humulone, a lipophilic constituent of hops that can be supercritically extracted, is a powerful and selective inhibitor of the inflammatory enzyme cyclooxygenase-2 (COX-2). Arthritis prescriptions such as Celebrex and Vioxx selectively inhibit COX-2. Research from two Japanese medical schools published in the *Journal of the Federation of European Bio-*

*chemical Societies* demonstrated that humulone also strongly inhibits COX-2. Hops may also inhibit or prevent Alzheimer's disease and colon cancer.

## $$ Horse Chestnut

Horse chestnut seed extract has been used in Germany for the last 200 years. Horse chestnut seeds *(Aesculus hippocastanum)* contain a complex mix of flavonols, including quercetin, kaempferol, rutin, and aescin. The flavonols function to increase the tone of the veins, thereby improving blood flow and to improve capillary integrity. Capillaries become excessively permeable when clot formation or excess pressure destroys some of the capillary wall. This results in increased permeability and facilitates the passage of minerals, proteins, and water through the walls, thereby producing swelling. The product works by decreasing transcapillary filtration, thus improving edema-related symptoms in venous disease of the legs. The product is available at health food stores as a capsule containing 600 mg. and 500 mg. aescin. Aescin is believed to exert anti-inflammatory properties, as well as decrease capillary permeability. It reduces the number and size of the small pores of the capillary wall, thus restricting water from leaving the capillaries. Additionally, more rutin is sometimes added to further decrease capillary fragility and restore normal permeability. In other products, vitamin E is also supplemented to reduce tissue oxidation.

## $$ Kava Kava

Kava root is used to calm body and mind and thwart insomnia. It improves low mood, muscle spasms uptightness and anxiety. Kava's relaxant properties are related to the lipid-like compounds known as lactones or pyrones. Researchers have identified six major kavalactones (a class of lactones) and another dozen minor ones. Like Valium and Xanax, they may influence GABA, the neurotransmitter that acts as a brake on the central nervous system.

It is supplied in capsules, liquids, and standardized extracts; a few sources offer dried kava in root pieces, cut and sifted and as a powder. For a mildly relaxing, anxiety-relieving effect, an average dose is 200 to 250mg of an extract standardized for 25 to 25 percent kavalactones, the chemical constituent thought responsible for kava's benefits.

Kava is remarkably safe as a relaxant. Even regular moderate use of kava among Pacific peoples seems to have no noticeable adverse effects on long-term health. Even transient side effects, such as mild nausea, are rare. High doses of potent kava products, however, can reduce one's motor control and lead to accidents, including fatal ones if one unwisely attempts to drive or operate heavy equipment after taking it. Persistent heavy consumption of kava may cause diarrhea, an overall lethargy and apathy or a scaly skin condition. Eliminating or cutting back on kava consumption reverses these conditions. Consuming too much or taking it in a strong tea causes numbness of the tongue.

**$$ Lactoferrin** (a non-herb and should be in supplement section)

Lactoferrin is produced from milk. All milk contains two major proteins, casein and whey. The latter is made up of peptides, a protein subfraction. Lactoferrin is one of these. In cows milk, less than one percent of whey protein is lactoferrin compared to mother's milk, which contains twelve percent! It is this subfraction that has documentation in the research literature to be antiviral, antibacterial, anticancer, and immune enhancing. Additionally, the apolactoferrin form, an iron depleted subtype, has the benefit of Lactoferrin plus acting as an antioxidant. Lactoferrin is found in micro concentrations in most other secretions such as saliva, tears, bronchial nasal, bile and pancreatic fluids. Modern filtering techniques have improved vastly in the last decade that we now have the technology to isolate large quantities of this unique substance from milk. Lactoferrin is not quite accepted by mainstream medicine. A recent study done by the Japanese National Cancer Research Institute, published in *Mutat Ros* April 2000; 462: 227-233, showed this may prevent colon cancer. More research in America indicates that this peptide limits tissue auto destruction and presents a new alternative for the future management for systemic inflammatory disease, such as rheumatoid arthritis. In that lactoferrin stimulates healthy intestinal cell growth as well as to enhance the growth of a friendly intestinal flora, it is a super probiotic. Apolactoferrin can be obtained from the Life Extension Foundation in sixty 300mg capsules for $30 and the dose is one capsule daily. Call 1/800/544-4440 or online at www.lif.org.

## $ Licorice

The herb's natural sweetness and flavor (it is fifty times sweeter than sugar) are due to its high content of glycyrrhizin. Glycyrrhizin is also responsible for most of licorice's medicinal properties, including its ability to reduce inflammation, especially in the gut, soothe throat tissues and reduce allergy symptoms. The ulcer-healing compounds in licorice are thought to be flavonoids. They apparently work by promoting the overall health of the gastrointestinal system rather than reducing the secretion of stomach acid that triggers ulcers. Additional compounds with therapeutic effects include sterols and gums.

Retailers sell licorice as a candy or in powders, capsules, lozenges, concentrated drops, tinctures and extracts. Chewable tablets and other licorice products for extended anti-ulcer therapy now often contain very little (just 2 percent or less) of the active component glycyrrhizin (also known as glycyrrhizic acid). These deglycyrrhizinated licorice (DGL) products cause fewer side effects and are much safer for long-term use than glycyrrhizin-containing licorice. An average dose of DGL licorice is 200mg.

Taking high or repeated doses of licorice extracts containing glycyrrhizin may cause adverse health by causing salt and water retention (including elevated blood pressure and low potassium). Avoid regular use of glycyrrhizin containing licorice products. These are tasteful and extremely safe.

## $$ Milk Thistle

Many people take milk thistle regularly to protect their liver from the effects of alcohol, heavy metals and drugs, and as needed after exposure to solvents, pesticides, bacteria from food poisoning or other toxins. Studies since the 1930s, conducted mainly in Germany, researched that the silymarin found in the herb works to stabilize liver cell membranes and act as an antioxidant to protect liver cells from free radical damage. It also helps regenerate healthy liver cells and boost the organ's ability to filter toxins from the blood. Researchers found that the antioxidant activity of a milk thistle seed extract reduced the liver damage typically seen in patients who take prescription anti-psychotic drugs for extended periods and particularly in death cap mushroom poisoning.

Milk thistle comes in capsules, liquids and teas; silymarin (the chemical constituent thought to be responsible for milk thistle's medical benefits) does not dissolve well in water, so the teas are very weak. The most popular products are standardized extracts of silymarin. An average dose is 200mg of an extract standardized for 70-80 percent silymarin calculated as oilybin. There are no side effects and contraindications. In fact, the plant's young (non-spiny) leaves and stems were once consumed as food in Europe. The plant contains B-sistosterol and is a similar ingredient in Take Control and Benecol. It thus lowers cholesterol and may help in a large prostate.

## $ Rosemary

Rosemary's *(Rosmarinus officinalis)* spiky, evergreen-like leaves contain flavonoids that have antioxidant properties. In fact, this tasty herb's antioxidant power was used for centuries to preserve food. One flavonoid in rosemary, diosmin, is reported to help strengthen capillaries, which can ease problems such as varicose veins and hemorrhoids.

Can rosemary help you stay young? In 1995, Japanese researchers found that two compounds in the herb, carnosol and carnosic acid, may help to protect body tissue and cells against the oxidative stresses that have been linked to diabete, aging, and coronary arteriosclerosis. So feel free to liberally spike your lamb, chicken, or roasted veggies with rosemary. It was voted as herb of the year in 2000 by the National Herb Association.

The German Commission E, the world's leading authority on herbs, has given the nod to using rosemary for circulation problems, such as low blood pressure, and for painful joints or muschles. Rosemary is often taken as a tea made from 1 teaspoon of the dried leaves per cup of water. To make tea using fresh leaves, double or triple the amount.

## $ Sage

Sage *(Salvia officianalis)* also acts as an effective antioxidant. Additionally, Commission E approves its internal use for indigestion and excessive perspiration. In fact, many traditional herbalists recommend sage tea as a remedy for menopausal night sweats. Commission E also approves sage as a gargle for throat irritations. It may be drunk as a tea, used as an extract or just a food seasoning. Some people report irritation and dryness of the mouth after consuming sage tea, so be cautious about using it too frequently.

## $ St. John's Wart

Well-controlled research show that St. John's Wart alleviates symptoms of depression, particularly seasoned effective disorders (SAD). In addition, it has been used as a topical arthritic wound and burn healer and an oral remedy to treat various viral conditions. Studies show that it is sedative and has anxious properties.

St. John's Wart is usually sold dried and in concentrated drops, tinctures and extracts. Its antidepressant effects may not be apparent until it is taken daily for three to four weeks. An average dose of a standardized extract containing 0.3 percent hypericin is 200 to 300mg.

The most common side effects from taking St. John's Wart are mild nausea, stomach ache, lack of appetite and tiredness, although these are not common. A very small percentage of people taking high daily doses of St. John's Wart may experience increased sensitivity to sunlight. Very remotely with a group of antidepressed, known as SSRI, like Prozac an serotenergic syndrome could occur characterized by confusion, tremors and sweating. In Lancet (February 12, 2000) there were two reports of how one of the constitutes of St. Johns Wart, the naphtodiantrons induce the liver isoenzyme of CYP3A4 and interfered with an intestinal drug transporter (p-glycoprotein). Both of these mechanisms caused a decrease of the availability of the cyclosporin, digoxin, dexamethasone (a cortisone drug), Propulsid, Cozar, Theoplyline, and Coumadin. Additionally, another report indicated the new AIDS drug, Indinavir, had less than an adequate blood level in patients taking St. Johns Wart. Since the liver cytochrome CYP3A4 and its intestinal counter part plays such a role in many drugs (statins, antibiotics), I suspect much more reports will be in the literature by the time you are reading this book. So "let the buyer beware" of St. Johns Wart, if they are taking other drugs. Unfortunately, your physician may not know about these interactions.

## $$ Sambucol

Sambucol is a powerful natural extract made from elderberry (see page 190), a plant long known for its remarkable ability to cure colds and flu. What is so exciting about Sambucol is its extraordinary success at *inactivating viruses*. Proven antiviral compounds are rare, especially natural ones. Research shows that Sambucol works by intercepting the viruses before they penetrate healthy cells. It has been used on seven different strains of new influenza viruses and proved effective on each one.

Sambucol was tested on actual patients during the massive Israeli flu epidemic of 1992-93. The results were spectacular. Within 24 hours, 20% of patients all had dramatic improvements in their symptoms. Bu the second day, 73% were improved. By day three, the figure jumped to 90%. *If Sambucol is taken at the first sign of flu, the problem should disappear within 24 to 48 hours.*

### $$$ Saw Palmetto

Saw Palmetto has become the premier herbal remedy for benign prostatic hypertrophy (BPH) symptoms, including discomfort and excessive nighttime and daytime urination. Saw Palmetto contains a number of compounds with potential therapeutic effects. Researchers have not yet identified with certainty the BPH related compounds, although the evidence points to B-sistosterol and fatty acids with an enzyme or hormone-related effect. For possible symptoms, it takes two months to work, although some of my patients claim overnight success. It also improves libido.

Saw Palmetto is supplied in liquid and standardized extract; it is frequently combined with pygeum *(Pygeum africanum),* stinging nettle, and pumpkin seed. Although Saw Palmetto is also available as a tea, the fatty acids in the herb thought to be at least partly responsible for its effects are not extracted well into water; thus, drinking a tea would not be as effective against BPH. The dose of Saw Palmetto is 160-320 mg of an extract standardized for 85 to 95 percent fatty acids and sterols. In rare cases nausea does occur.

No long-term toxicity has been reported. Frequently added to it with the other herbs is zinc in a combination capsule. Recently, B-sitosterol found in the herb, a similar product to B-sitostanol, in Benecol and Take Control (see page 79) is a much better source and less expensive than the herb. It also helps with lowering the cholesterol.

### $$ Siberian Ginseng

It supports the working of the adrenal glands and helps with nervous tension. It tends to increase energy, extend endurance and fight fatigue. Siberian Ginseng also boosts overall immune function and may play a role in the treatment of hypertension, blood sugar irregularities and depression. Siberian Ginseng remedies are derived from the roots and sometimes from the leaves. Studies on Siberian Ginseng have shown that it has considerable promise for increasing longevity and improving overall health. Chemists have isolated more than three dozen compounds in Siberian Ginseng that may affect the mind and body; foremost among these are the eleutherosides, which occur in the plant's roots and, to a lesser degree, in the leaves. Studies have determined that the eleutherosides differ form the ginsenosides isolated from the panax ginsengs, though some of their effects on the body are similar. Exactly how these compounds affect the body is still being determined. The effects, in fact, may be available only from the whole herb. The isolated components of Siberian Ginseng do not have the same tonic action as the whole plant. In a recent study on experienced distance runners, researchers saw no effects on exercise performance with the extract.

Siberian Ginseng is sold in capsules, tinctures, and extracts. Standardized Siberian Ginseng products often specify the content of one or more of a series of chemicals known as eleutherosides. An average dose is 100mg of an extract standardized for one percent eleutherosides.

Siberian Ginseng is considered to be safe for daily consumption even in doses many times larger than average, though some people may experience insomnia and other side effects from taking high amounts.

### $ Silver (should be in the mineral section)

Silver has been used since antiquity for its healing and preserving powers. The ancient Greeks kept their medicinal liquids (and expensive foods) free of contamination by placing them in the silver jars. Since the middle ages, silver was a stable for cooking and eating with silver pans, plates, and utensils. Our grandparents perhaps had less illness because of ingesting minute particles of silver from these. Silver and its salt have been used for centuries for disease treatment, one hundred-fifty years ago for syphilis, in the last one hundred years for eye and nose drops, gargles, douches, and the last 30 years topically for burn victims by mainstream physicians.

Silver has been proven toxic to all species of bacteria, protozoa, parasites, and many viruses. It acts as a toxin in one-celled organisms, disabling several enzyme systems needed for their existence. Mammals do not have these metabolic pathways and therefore it does not harm our tissue. *Movidyn,* a powdered form of colloidal silver, is a discovery of the previous Soviet Union in the '60s was not only used as a super disinfectant but was offered as a counter agent against germ warfare. There is a correlation between low human levels of silver and sickness, to include even cancer. Currently silver is used in home water filters, airline water systems, and progressive community water companies for its antibacterial purifying effect.

Today silver is made in ultramicroscopic particles in a colloidal solution suspended in deionized water by electromagnetic charges. This ultra fine 99.999% silver has a particle size from 0.0001 to 0.001 microns. A red blood cell is a giant compared to this being 7 microns or 7 million times bigger! After ingestion, this metal enters the blood stream within 20 minutes and of course goes where the blood goes, i.e., all over our body. Colloidal silver can be obtained for less than $2 an ounce at health food stores. Or with equipment costing less than $100, one can make gallons of it for $5. Since it is light sensitive, it should be kept in darkly tinted glass bottles in a cool place. Plastic containers magnetize easily and the silver particles will stick to the sides. Also keep it away from magnetic fields such as electronics or motors since they too will interfere with the ions, holding the colloid in solution. If placed in the refrigerator, the silver may fall out of solution. Colloidal silver is predictably safe. As a pre-1938 medicinal it is out of the control of the FDA. There is a rare benign state referred to as argyria of which I have not been seen in the thirty years due to the ingestion of too much silver over decades in which the skin turns blue. I recommend several ounces of 5 to 100 ppm for ingestion and up to 500 ppm for topical use.

## $$ Stinging Nettle
This has been used for over 200 years in Germany particularly for inflammatory conditions, such as arthritis. In

the last 50 years it has been used additionally for allergies to include hay fever. Research has shown that it does boost our immunity and as such is a vitalizing nutrient and plays a role in both cancer and infection. It also has been used as a prevention for symptoms of prostate enlargement similar to saw palmetto (see page 207). The extract of the herb has been used externally for oily hair and scalp and the treatment of dandruff. In this country it is available in tinctures and capsules. Follow the directions on the label.

## $ Valerian

Valerian is effective in promoting sleep, relaxes mind and body, provides temporary relief from anxiety, and calms a nervous stomach. It can also help relieve headaches, menstrual cramps and constipation or indigestion from nervous tension. Many extracts are now standardized for valerenic acid, which may interact with receptors for GABA, the calming brain chemical. Valerian is supplied in tinctures and extracts; it is frequently combined with other calming herbs (kava kava, chamomile, skull cap, passion flower) in natural insomnia remedies. Valerian root has an unpleasant smell, reminiscent of a pair of rotten socks and cats love the smell, so many people prefer the less odorific capsules to liquid remedies. An average dose is 100 to 200mg of valerian extract standardized to contain 0.8 to 1.0 percent valerenic acid, a compound that occurs in the root. It works almost immediately. Side effects are minimal. Valerian is much safer than prescription sedatives. However, as with any relaxant, one should not take it before doing tasks that require full alertness, nor should one use it regularly for an extended period of time (more than a few weeks). A small minority may find valerian stimulating instead of calming.

## $$ Yohimbine

The anti-aging benefits of yohimbine are improvement of strength and duration, as well as improved sexual performance, paricularly due to erectile dysfunction. Rarely, Yohimbine can lead to over stimulation to the point of nervousness and anxiety. Other side effects may include nausea, vomiting, increased blood pressure, tremors, dizziness and headaches.

Yohimbine is available in 1mg, 2.5mg, 3.75mg, 5mg and 10mg tablets under the trade names such as Aphrodyne and Viengra. Doses of more than 2.5mg require a prescription. It is frequently combined with other products.

## IV. OTHER SUPPLEMENTS

### $ Acetaminophen

Although we've known for over thirty years that aspirin does "thin the blood" by decreasing the activity of platelets, the small cellular elements in the blood that cause clotting. Its first cousin, acetaminophen (Tylenol) has been shown to work in conjunction with the aspirin. At the University of Georgia, Dr. Phillip Greenspan found that the acetaminophen is a potent inhibitor of the enzyme, myeloperoxidase. This enzyme oxidizes the LDL, modifies it in such a way that it is more delectable to the certain white cells that reside within the wall of our arteries. It is the cells, which we call macrophages that ingest the LDL cholesterol and cause the plaque and obstruction, atherosclerosis. In that the acetaminophen blocks the activity of this enzyme, there is less transformation of the bad cholesterol (LDL) that is available for the macrophages to ingest. Although the dose of the acetaminophen has not been worked out, I would suggest taking one extra strength Tylenol (500 mg) or its generic equivalent twice a day. This research was presented at the conference on arteriosclerosis, thrombosis and vascular biology in Denver, May 21, 2000. It may be wise to take two adult aspirin once a month, a child's aspirin every day thereafter and every day of the month, with two extra strength generic Tylenol (acetaminophen). The Tylenol is complimentary to the aspirin. This can also be taken to prevent pain. Some people state it helps them to sleep, and one is welcome to take it at bedtime.

This program should cost less than ten cents a day and is well worth the price.

### $$$ Acetyl-L-Cartninine (ALC)

An occurring nutrient naturally in our body, ALC transports fats into the ,mitochondria, the micro energy producers in our cells. It is found in many common foods to include milk. ALC helps protect the brain by nourishing its receptors, which normally decline with age. ALC also prevents the formation of lipofuscin, an age pigment, and improves cerebral blood flow. ALC's anti-aging benefits are decreasing brain aging, improving memory, and increasing concentration. It is helpful in Alzheimer's disease, and is used as a "smart drug" (makes us smarter).

Side effects are rare. Nausea, headache, dizziness or vomiting can occur when starting treatment and at high dosages (greater than 1500mg/d). ALC is supplied in 250mg and 500mg tablets, as well as a liquid form. Pharmaceutical trade name preparations include Branigen, Ceredor, Nicetile, Normobren and Zibren. It is frequently taken with carnitine (see page 220).

### $$$$ Adrafinil (Modafinil)

Adrafinil stimulates brain activity. Modafinil, which is similar but even more potent, is more expensive. Both drugs act on receptors, making them more susceptible to norepinephrine. This increases alertness, concentration, and short term memory, and improves hand/eye coordination. Adrafinil is an alpha-adrenergic agonist chemically almost identical to Modafinil.

Side effects are abuse and drug interactions, and therefore usage should be monitored by a knowledgable physician. Modanfil is listed as a Schedule IV of the Controlled Substances Act. People with epilepsy, liver or kidney impairment, or those using tranquilizers should avoid Adrafinil and Modafinil. Caution is advised if used in combination with norepinephrine-stimulating agents such as Yohimbine. Adrafinil is supplied in 300mg tablets under the trade name

Olmifon 300 to 1500mg. Modafinil is supplied under the trade name Provigil™ in 100 and 200mg tablets, and 200 to 400mg a day is the usual dose.

### $$$$ Aminoguanidine

Gylcosylation (see box at the end of this product) is the pathological binding of glucose to an amino acid that results in the formation of a non-functioning structure in the tissue. Diabetics suffer from an accelerated rate of glycosylation, and many of the premature degenerative diseases common in Type I and Type II diabetes is attributed to the glycosylation process. As organisms age, glycosylation becomes a major factor in the development of age-related disease. Some gerontologists believe that glycosylation is the most significant biologic event responsible for the degenerative diseases of the eye, arteries, and the brain. Those seeking to add healthy years to their lives have a significant interest in interfering with the glycosylation process. Oxidative damage plays a role in the glycosylation process, which helps to explain why antioxidant supplements have shown benefit in preventing these diseases. It requires a lot more than antioxidant, however, to adequately block age-related glycosylation.

While a number of anti-glycating agents are in the development stage, aminoguanidine has been available in Europe for many years. Healthy adults may consider taking 300 mg of aminoguanidine a day (or every other day), while diabetics could consider a maximum dose of 600 mg a day. Semi-monthly blood tests should be considered in order to protect against any unknown toxicities.

As more European suppliers have begun offering aminoguanidine, the cost has declined sharply, making this a reasonable addition to one's life extension regimen. For a free directory of offshore suppliers offering aminoguanidine to Americans for personal use, write to International Society for Free Choice, 9 Dubnov Street, 64368 Tel Aviv, Israel.

**Glycosylation** is an enzymatic process by which sugars are attached to proteins-although the term "non-enzymatic glycosylation" is commonly used. "Glycation" is the better word that is used to describe the non-enzymatic attachment of sugars to proteins. Glycosylation is reversible, wheras glycation is either irreversible, or leads to Advanced Glycation End-products (AGEs). This protein cross-linking is characteristic of long-live proteins and is notable for malfunction of many organs. It is likened to "rusting" of tissue and contributes to the aging process.

### $ (L) Arginine

L-Arginine (pronounced el-AR-ji-neen) is a naturally occuring amino acid. This has received favorable reports in preventing and treating heart disease, cancer and infection. It works as a precursor for endothelial cell releasing factor (ECRF), or now thought to be nitric oxide. This is a substance produced by one's own blood vessels that keeps the blood vessel open (vasodilatation) rather than spastically closed (vasoconstriction), dilating the coronary and other arteries. It may prevent angina (chest pain due to coronary vasoconstriction) or a heart attack. Working on the peripheral arterioles, it is used to treat or prevent heart failure (the inability of the heart as a pump to keep up with the bodily needs of supply). It has been exceedingly helpful in peripheral arterial disease in which the leg does not get enough blood for the exercising muscle. This results in leg cramps, a condition that L-Arginine even prevents the build up of cholesterol plaque and clot within all of our blood vessels. It also is a great adjunct for erectile dysfunction.

Arginine may help release our growth hormone, the naturally rejuvenating hormone. It also may promote sexual function, keep blood pressure normalized, improve coordination and long term memory and enhance our sense of smell. In the *European Journal of Nutrition* (27:690-695,'97), arginine might improve insulin sensitivity in Syndrome X and *Type II Diabetes*. It also is a free radical scavenger, not only internally but externally, thus causing an anti-aging effect on the skin and the internal organs. Additionally, L-Arginine has been shown to stimulate the immune function in several animal studies. It has been used in combination with traditional approaches for the treatment of cancer, particularly cancer of the breast. In an article from The University of Minnesota, oral L-Arginine in doses of 3gm twice a day taken with meals was recommended.

Although we get 5 to 6gm of this natural chemical in our food such as meat (including chicken) and nuts, to do the job we need an additional 6gm. This is an extremely safe product and the only side effect ever described in an overdose of L-Arginine was mild diarrhea. It is best to split the dose into 3 gm twice a day. Some doctors recommend even up to 12 gm a day. L-Arginine is supplied in 500 mg and 1,000 mg capsules as well as a powder (1 teaspoon equals 4,000 mg) and bars.

Twin Lab sells 100 capsules of 500 mg each for $14.00. It is recommended taking six capsules of 1,000mg each for $11.00, or 65 cents daily. Heart Bars sold in super markets, health food stores and pharmacies have over 3 gm of L-Arginine in each (as well as other heart healthy nutrients such as vitamins $B_{12}$, C, E, folic acid, niacin and soy porducts). From Life Enhancement (1-800-543-3873); www.lifeenhancement.-com other products with arginine include Inner Power, ProSexual Plus, Male Befor and After Glow, Virca Clear, and Living Skin.

### $ Aspirin

Aspirin prevents the platelets to clot in the blood, be it in the heart vessels which can cause a heart attack, or in the neck and head vessels which can cause a stroke. The basis for the use of low dose aspirin lies in its unique inhibitory effect on a single key enzyme. This is COX-1 (cyclooxygenase-1). Actually, there are two forms (isoform) of COX. The other is known as COX-2. The latter is inducible and undetectable in most normal tissues but under certain conditions such as inflammatory processes, becomes elevated. Therefore, a high dose of aspirin (10 grains or 2 adult tablets), which is an anti-inflammatory and other medications such as ibuprofen quell the COX-2 and the inflammatory process. As a consequence of this, the good effects of COX-2, which gives protection of the stomach and kidneys are lost and problems with this such as ulcers, gastrointestinal bleeding, kidney failure, fluid retention and high blood pressure are lost with the higher dosage.

Aspirin is absorbed and goes directly to the liver. The liver inactivates the aspirin by deacetylation. A transdermal patch may be available soon that will not do this, in that it would go right into the blood stream to do its good thing of preventing excess blood clotting. Aspirin has also been shown to decrease the incidence of gastrointestinal cancer and gall bladder disease, and improve diabetes, PMS symptoms, and pregnancy outcomes. The American Cancer Society epidemiologists found that while low dose aspirin use had no effect on cancers of most organ systems, the risks were greatly reduced for fatal cancers of the esophagus, stomach, rectum and colon. These four digestive tract cancers were approximately 40% lower among men and women who used aspirin 16 times per month or more for at least one year compared to those who used no aspirin. As mentioned, aspirin prevents gall bladder disease.

When cholesterol-saturated bile accumulates and becomes thicken, it slows down the flow in the large bile channel, and gallstones are formed. During acute inflammation, usually a bacterial infection associated with gallstones, the production of prostaglandins are increased as part of the normal inflammation and repair processes. This process involves much pain, increased fluid secretions, muscle contraction and decreased bile, all of which perpetuate the inflammation more. Several studies have been conducted to show that prostaglandin inhibitors such as aspirin and non-steroidal anti-inflammatory drugs can prevent the formation of gallstones, as well as reduce the biliary pain associated with this process.

Years ago researchers noticed a link between arthritis, leprosy and the incidence of Alzheimer's. As part of the standard treatment for arthritis and leprosy was the use of aspirin. These patients were proven to have a lower incidence of Alzheimer's. Researchers from Johns Hopkins Alzheimer's Disease Research Center found that as the use of aspirin and other non-steroidal anti-inflammatory drugs increases, the rate of mental deterioration decreases. In the November 8, 1999 issue of *Business Week*, a pharmaceutical report indicated anti-inflammatory drugs reduce the inflammation that accompanies plaque formation in the brain. Also, population studies have long noted that aspirin and other non-steroidal anti-inflammatory drugs appear to reduce the risk of Alzheimer's by 50%."

In diabetes and borderline diabetes, aspirin magnifies and enhances the effects of insulin and oral hypoglycemic agents. So aspirin may protect somewhat diabetic risk. Many small studies have concluded that low dose aspirin reduces the risks of pregnancy induced hypertension toxcemia and severe low birth weight.

I do recommend enteric coated aspirin, such as 81 mg Bayer, (120 count) or a generic variety compared to the child's aspirin, which are in a tamper-proof bottle with a count of only 20 or so. When one does need an analgesic please read the label to make sure you do not take a product that contains additional aspirin. Acetaminophen (generic Tylenol) certainly is a good substitute.

There is some controversy in that some doctors feel that a higher dose of aspirin may be of benefit. I do compromise and suggest the first day of each month, a person would take two adult (325mg) aspirin, or if they don't have them, 8 of the child's aspirin and the every day of the month thereafter take one child's aspirin.

### $$$ Astaxanthin

Astaxanthin is one of the natural carotenoids found mainly in algae, particularly *Haemococcus Plusvialis*. It gives the pink color to salmon, shrimp, and flamingos, all of which live in marine environments and obtain this chemical either directly, or indirectly such as eating insects, which have ingested this algae. Claims for this product include antioxidation, improvement of the immune system, anti-inflammatory, lipid improvement, and cancer prevention. Unlike beta carotene and most other carotenoids, astaxanthine crosses the blood retinal/brain barrier offering protection for macular degeneration. This agent raises the good (HDL) cholesterol. Also, it antagonizes a wide range of cancer promoters and in particular has been shown to decrease the size of cancer of the colon, liver, oral cavity, and bladder. Astaxanthin is not a precursor of vitamin A, and therefore even in large doses it does not cause toxicity. It is synthesized by lower organisms through a series of intermediates such as canthaxanthin and lycopene and may be metabolized by our bodies to some of these important antioxidants. As an antioxidant, it alone milligram for milligram has 100 times the power of vitamin E. The recommended dosage is 2 to 4 mg. per day and can be obtained in IMS capsules from LAHAYE over their website: www.lahaye.com.

### $$$ Beta Glucan

Beta glucan is a type of polysaccharide found in a variety of substances such as oats, barley, mushrooms, and fungi. Beta glucans activate vital components of the immune system, specifically the macrophage. Beta glucan, defined technically as *B*-1, 3/2,6 glucans, is a macro molecule with glucose molecules linked in so-called *B*-1,3 positions. The degree of branching present in the Beta 1,3/1,6 Glucan molecule determines the level of activity. Beta Glucan found in oats and barley have little or no activity. Beta glucan found in mushrooms contain branching with only single glucose molecules and produce only a certain degree of immune enhancing activity. On the other hand,

Beta Glucan extracted from baker's yeast *(Saccharomyces Cerevisiae)* cell wall contains very extensive branching and is capable of producing the most powerful immune enhancing activity of all Beta Glucans. These cells activated by Beta 1,3/1,6 Glucan become more alert, better able to engulf, kill and digest invading microorganism, and also secrete signal molecules called cytokines which stimulate the production of new white blood cells and simultaneously make the antibody producing cells more active. The brand name of Beta 1,3/1,6 Glucan is IMMUTAL™. The manufacturer suggests a month loading dose of IMMUTAL™ 425 to be followed with a dose of IMMUTAL™ 100. It is available at A.T.I.N., 1582 W. Deere Ave., Suite C, Dept. 400, Irvine, CA 92606. Or call them TOLL FREE at: 1/800/446-3063, Ext. 400.

## $$ Bromelain

Bromelain from pineapple has a mild, soothing effect on the stomach and aids in protein digestion. Also, it is an anti-inflammatory enzyme useful in post traumatic responses with swelling and after surgery in that it reduces tissue irritation. This enzyme has several actions that make it helpful in the prevention and treatment of cardiovascular disease. It reduces platelet aggregation, arterial plaquing, and clot formation. This product has been shown to reduce the symptoms of angina pectoris. Another popular use has been to reduce joint inflammation in rheumatoid arthritis. The ranges for bromclain's anti-inflammatory effects appear to be from 500-2,000 mg. daily, usually taken in two doses. A potential medical use of this enzyme as well as others collectively do clear the blood of large particles that are noticed in live blood analysis and may clog up small capillaries impairing tissue nourishment. Bromelain is very inexpensive and can be purchased at any health food store.

## $$ Carnitine

If one is on a low-fat diet, they may not be getting another important heart nutrient, carnitine, which is found mainly in red meat. The primary function of carnitine is to escort fatty acids to the furnace (cell mitochondria), where the fat is burned to produce energy. In doing so, it reduces the fat levels in the blood dramatically. Johns Hopkins Medical Journal reported that carnitine lowers bad cholesterol and raises the good. Dr. Carl Pepine of the Division of Cardiology at University of Florida Medical School indicated that tests show carnitine increased blood flow in the heart by 60 percent and reduced vascular resistance by 25 percent. Taken with antioxidants such as lipoic acid and coenzyme Q10 plus the Omega 3's (fish oil) it speeds up the metabolism of fat, causes weight loss and allows our cells to function even under conditions of decreased oxygen. Alone it improves life expectency with coronary artery disease and congestive heart failure.

As we age, our mitochondrial engine functions less efficiently and produces less chemical energy (ATP). The minimal energy is directed toward survival processes such as chemical transport rather than cell repair, immune functions, and tissue building. Carnitine is a water soluble vitamin-like compound. Similar to choline and other B vitamins, it turns food stuff into energy. Humans can synthesize a small amount of the body's needs of carnitine (less than 25%) from the amino acid lysine. The rest come from diet (meat, fish, eggs, cheese) and supplements.

There are no side effects of carnitine. It is supplied in tablets of 500 to 1,000mg as well as powder (1 teaspoon equals 4,000mg). Between 1 gram (1,000mg) and 4 grams a day is the usual dose. This should be taken in the morning and for better result take together with acetyl –L carnitine (ALC) 500 to 1,500mg. (See page 212 for information on ALC).

## $$$$ Centrophenoxine

This removes lipofuscin, an age pigment from the brain, heart and skin. Appearances of lipofuscin in the skin are referred to as liver spot. It also increases certain brain protein and helps the brain cell metabolism. The anti-aging benefits include protection against free radical damage, increased mental energy, improved memory, and prevention and treatment of stroke and brain injury. Possible side effects_include nausea or mild dizziness. People with severely high blood pressure or epilepsy should avoid this supplement. Centrophenoxine is supplied in 250mg-tablet form under the trade names Cerutil, Helfergin and Lucidril. It works similar, but better than its sister chemical DMAE.

## $$ Cetyl Myristoleate (CMO)

Derived from fat found in beavers, albino mice, and sperm whales, CMO functions as a surfactant, or lubricant, to loosen tight joints and tissues. CMO might even lubricate ones arteries. Also, this product may work for patients for whom nonsteroidal anti-inflammatory drugs and corticosteroids have not been effective. CMO has no adverse side effects, in contrast to NSAIDs, which has a high incidence. More than that, cetyl myristoleate may help calm hyperimmune responses and regulate immune systems that are not working at optimal level, thus benefiting those suffering from autoimmune diseases such as multiple sclerosis, lupus, and rheumatoid arthritis. Reputedly patients with fibromyalgia and chronic fatigue syndrome have benefited from CMO.

The discovery of cetyl myristoleate began in 1962, when research scientist Dr. Harry Diehl from the National Institutes of Health was given an assignment to create arthritis in a certain group of mice to test a new arthritis drug. Because an injection of Freund's adjuvant induces arthritic symptoms in most animals, Dr. Diehl proceeded to inject Swiss Albino mice, but discovered that these mice did not develop arthritis. What did the Swiss Albino mouse have in its body that prevented it from getting arthritis? Dr. Diehl worked on this project for two years, and in 1964 he isolated a substance that was unique to this particular mouse strain. It turned out to be a fatty acid ester that we now know as cetyl myristoleate.

CMO is a naturally occurring fatty acid ester. It works as a natural anti-inflammatory in diseases such as arthritis, tendonitis, bursitis, etc. The product also helps modulate immune system function (apparently by inhibiting leukotriene B4 and manipulating prostaglandin metabolism), making it effective in treating autoimmune diseases such as lupus and rheumatoid arthritis. CMO acts as a surfactant, or super lubricant, to improve the synovial fluid in our joints so they glide more easily and are less stiff. Indeed, relief of morning stiffness is often one of the first improvements that patients experience with cetyl myristoleate. Although I have no personal experience with the product, the improvement is quick, with an average of 80% clearly improving within two weeks. If local health food stores don't carry CMO, order it from Longevity Science at (800)933-9440. It is also available as Colastin™, which has other complimentary ingredients for the anti-aging and inflammation process from PNR (888)-737-7307. There is some concern that synehetically produced CMO has the TRANS type of fatty hydrogenated acid made from vegetable oils and could damage cellular membranes. An authentic product — Arth CMO — made from animal fat can be obtained from Frank Landig, 972/239-6901. Dr. Paul Barney, author of the *Doctor's Guide to Natural Medicine,* reports that, "tests which have been run on cetyl myristoleate containing products have found no side effect or toxicity."

### $$$ Colostrum

Historically, bovine colostrum has played a significant role in natural healing. It has been used in India for thousands of years. Ayurvedic physicians and the Rishis have documented colostrum's physical and spiritual benefits. They make a candy by dropping the colostrum in boiling water and then coating it with sugar. People in Scandinavia and northern European countries are very familiar with the healing benefits of colostrum. They make a delicious pudding dessert, topped with honey, to celebrate the birth of a calf and its good health. In the United States and throughout the world, bovine colostrum was used for immune purposes prior to the introductions of sulfa drugs and antibiotics. In the early 50's, Dr. Albert Sabin became aware of the possibilities of colostrum. He found these antibodies, grew them in a cultured media and produced the first antiviral vaccine.

Hundreds of years of human use, thousands of scientific studies and human clinical trials world-wide have shown bovine colostrum to be safe and effective. Colostrum is available without a prescription in health food stores. The freeze-dried preparation in capsules is what I recommend. Those in a compressed pill form may have change in molecular structure due to heat and pressure and will have loss some of its potency.

### $$$$ Conjunctisana

This is used specifically to treat degeneration, near sightedness, and macular degeneration. This product which is a concoction- of bovine origin has organ factors from corresponding cow eye tissue. Each liquid capsule contains; 0.2ng bulb.oc. fet., 0.05ng lenx, 0.1ng fet. Vessels, 0.15ng placenta fet., 0.05pg retina, 0.05pg optic nerve, 0.lpg choriod, 0.lpg hyaloid body, 0.05pg cerebral cortx, 0.05pg diencephalon as well as the pharmaceutical substances 0.074ug deslanoside C, 5ug aesulin and 5ug sodium dodecyl sulfate, 4 percent glycerol ad 0.5ml saline (0.7 percent). There are known side effects or contraindications. VitOrgan of Germany is supplied by Conjunctisan A in 0.5 ml liquid droppers and can be purchased in health food stores.

### $ Creatinine

Another supplement worthy of consideration is creatinine monohydrate, which really is an ergogenic. Usually, it comes from both our diet and our production. Creatinine is produced in our body's liver, pancreas and kidneys and is part of our body's energy cycle. It increases our intramuscular levels of creatinine phosphate, a high energy coumpound. It figures into the high-energy phosphate (ATP) used in most metabolic reactions in voluntary as well as involuntary movement. Muscle builders use this to build bulk in muscles as well as to make them lift still heavier weights. Aerobic athletes such as runners or bike riders benefit as well. However, in the normal individual, it can aid in work-outs, helping a person not only look, but perform better muscularly. Red meat contains creatinine, but also has some other undesirable substances (cholesterol and iron). Fish contains some creatinine but less than red meat. It can help to take 5 to 15 grams a day as a supplement. It is without *side effects,* rarely causing muscle cramping, which easily is combated by taking some extra magnesium.

### $$$$ Deprenyl

This is a drug that is used to treat Parkinson's disease. It's anti-aging benefits include improved memory, slowing of the loss of sexual capacity and increased life span. Side effects can include nausea, stomach ache, drowsiness and depression. High dosages can result in sudden high blood pressure and agitation. Standard dosage for humans is 10 mg/day. Deprenyl is sold in the U.S. for treatment of Parkinson's disease under the name Eldepryl and is fairly expensive. It does require a prescription.

### $ DMAE (Dimethylaminoethanol)

It is a cell membrane stabilizer and a precursor to acetylcholine. DMAE is closely related to DEAE (Diethylaminoethanol) in GH3. Gerovital $H_3$ or $GH_3$, an antiaging drug, was developed by Ana Aslan, M.D. To order call 1/800/GH3-2696. It removes lipofuscin (accumulation of toxic pigments) from tissue, including nerve and brain cells. DMAE improves free-radical scavenging of other antioxidants, increases life span, including maximum life span in experimental animals. Has extended life span of older animals. Used to enhance memory, it may be an adjunct in the treatment of Alzheimer's disease. It should be taken in the morning to avoid insomnia.

## $ Dihydroendosterone (DHEA)

DHEA is a naturally produced hormone by the adrenals. It peaks at approximately age 25 and then declines. The day it begins to decline is the day that an individual "starts dying." Studies have shown that when it falls to very low levels, the end is close for most individuals. There have been many studies done and some of the research shows that this DHEA may be an anti-aging product, and if used in physiologic doses, can retard this natural process of aging. In over 2,500 medical references regarding this substance, there are some excellent articles in the prevention of cancer, arteriosclerosis, autoimmune diseases such as lupus, chronic fatigue syndrome, Alzheimer's disease, hypercholesterolemia, depression and osteoporosis. It also helps sexual function and causes weight loss in the overweight patient and has been touted to reduce the sugar lowering mediations in diabetes. Under extreme stress, one needs more DHEA and at times I use it in younger acutely or chronically ill individuals. It comes form natural sources such as the Mexican yam (Dioscorea). I used to recommend a serum and /or sputum level of DHEA and then prescribe, if low. But *all* patients over age 40 had a lower level than a 25-year-old, the age we all should wish to be to have peak youth and health. I have stopped doing these studies. There may be some enhancement of the DHEA by other substance. Dr. V.M. Dilman reported recently in the Journal of Gerontology that chromium increased the life span of rats by an awesome 26 percent because of the increased production of DHEA. We have personally studied over 200 patients measuring DHEA levels and compared them with various proprietary preparation and found them all to have the active chemical. DHEA metabolizes to testosterone and estrogen, so the side effect is that regular DHEA could cause slight acne, facial hair and lower the voice when taken in high doses, and might increase the risk of prostate and breast cancer. Keto-DHEA may be a safer version in that it is not converted to sex hormones. Pharmaceutical grade of both products is readily available in pharmacies and health food stores without prescription. It is supplied in 5, 25, 50, and 75mg sice. I recommend 25 to 100mg a day, taken first thing in the morning with or without food. This can be taken with any other drug or supplement. Again, the lower ones DHEA, the less the longevity. The greater it is over 150, the longer you will live. This should improve not only the quantity of your life, but the quality as well.

## $$$ Estrogen

Estrogen are a class of hormones produced in the ovaries, or made from other hormones in fat cells. There are three estrogens: estradiol, estratiol and estrone. These natural hormones work more efficiently compared to synthetic estrogens or, even worse, animal estrogens. The most common animal product is Conjugated Equine Estrogen (Premarin™). The proper dose is titrated against the pituitary hormones of LH and FSH. These are prescription drugs, but soy products can act as a surrogate for estrogen. Although estrogen may be good for men, according to studies, I now recommend it only for women. Using estrogen alone in women, with their uterus still present, could, in a few percent, cause cancer of that organ. (See page 299 for further information on estrogen).

## $$ Fatty Acids (Activated)

For pain relief and easier movement, fish oil supplements are excellent. Fish oil provides us with two crucial, sorely needed omega-3 essential fats — EPA (eicosapentaenoic acid) and DHA (docosahexaenoic acid). The omega-3s are cornerstones for the body's many eicosanoids. These hormone-like chemicals are responsible for countless bodily functions, including causing and counteracting inflammation.

One particular omega-6 fat, gamma-linoleic acid (GLA), works in concert with EPA and DHA to cool inflammation. Found in borage oil, evening primrose oil, and black currant seeds, it's the principal building block for one of the most important eicosanoids, prostaglandin $E_1$. These oils are so important that some scientists refer to them as vitamin F (see page 159). Take 360-720 mg of EFA, 240-480 mg of DHA, and 1000-2000 mg of GLA every day.

#### $$$$ Glucosamine/Chondroitin Sulate

Glucosamine promotes the production of a special chemical called proteoglycans, which are water retaining molecules that are the building blocks of cartilage. Chondroitin Sulfate is the nutrient that blocks the enzymes that destroy cartilage. Depending on ones weight, I recommend taking between 1200mg of Glucosamine combined with 800-1600mg Chondroitin Sulfate. Various formulations exist with many other ingredients on the market. Used by me for the last decade for my patients, these compounds are now going mainstream (JAMA; 2000: 283; 1469-1474) and being recommended by many such physicians including the orthopedic specialist. Aflexa™ produced by McNeil, the makers of Tylenol™, is pure glucosamine, but at a lower dose than most preparations and without its helper chondrotin sulfate, this product may be more accessible to people but slightly inferior to the other products on the market at health food stores.

Taken early before arthritis begins, it may ward off this disease. The cartilage of cows and even more obtainable from chickens is loaded with proteoglycans similar to Glucosamine and Chodroitin. I have been munching the ends of chicken thighs and legs for the last 40 years.

#### $$$$ Glucarate (See page 197)

#### $$$ Glutamine

Glutamine is the most abundant amino acid found in the human body. It was once thought to be a non-essential amino acid. Now we consider this as a "conditionally essential amino acid". That is to say that, when people are under stress such as acute and chronic illness, psychological stress, or surgery, they do not have enough glutamine in the system. Glutamine, along with N-acytl cysteine forms the most important natural compound in our body, glutathione.It is also used to combat such diseases as Crohn's disease, irritable bowl disease, ulcerative colitis and lupus. It is an extremely safe nutrient with no side effects. I recommend 2 to 6 grams, taken in juice (it does come as a powder) in mid-afternoon. It will also act at that time as a "pick-me-up" tonic and a stimulation of the immune system.

## $$ 5-Hydroxytryptophan (5-HTP)

5-HTP is a naturally occuring substance derived from the seed pods of *Griffonia simplicifolia,* a West African medicinal plant. In humans, 5-HTP is the immediated nutrient precursor to the neurotransmitter serotonin (5-HTP). This means that 5-HTP converts directly into serotonin in the brain. Serotonin has many profoundly important functions, including a role in sleep, appetite, memory, learning, temperature regulation, mood, sexual behavior, cardiovascular function, muscle contraction, and endocrine regulation.

Serotonin production declines with age, and at any age its abundance can be compromised further by stress. Low levels of serotonin are most commonly manifested by depressed mood, anxiety, and insomnia. They can also lead to various other complaints and disorders, diminishing one's quality of life. Life can be improved by supplementing with 5-HTP. It can restore serotonin levels and help improve general mood, insomnia, chronic headaches, depression, weight loss, migraines, anxiety, PMS, and Fibromyalgia.

This is a safer form than the Tryptophan and is equally as effective. It doesn't require a prescription. Take 100 mg of 5-HTP 3x's a day. It comes in 25, 50 and 100 mg capsules.

## $$$$ Human Growth Hormone (HGH)

Growth Hormone is a misnomer. It should be called Antiaging Hormone. Its "legitimate" use is for pituitary dwarfed children, although a recent article in Lancet gives credence that it will render congenitally short statured children into normal size adults. First discovered in 1921, HGH was isolated in 1956 and over the ensuing three decades its 191 amino acid sequence has been worked out, first by Genentech in 1986 and later by several other drug companies using recombiant DNA techniques. Thus bio engineered growth hormone could be produced in vast quantities by special bacteria and recently by mamilian cells. Previously, it had to be harvested form cadavers and was abandoned in 1987, because of a contaminating virus causing disease in the recipient similar to Mad Cow Disease. The physiology of HGH is complex and the decline in production is age related. It is secreted by the pituitary gland and causes growth and repair of the body's tissue through several intermediate steps such as IGF-1.

## $$ Huperzine A

Huperzine A is another natural memory enhancer. It is an extract from the Chinese club moss and appears to maintain higher acetycholine levels by inhibiting acetycholinesterase, the enzyme that breaks down acetycholine. This seems to be a promising adjuvant agent in the treatment of Alzheimer's disease. Additionally, Huperzine A is a great short-term memory booster that can be taken in doses of 50 mcg to 100 mcg first thing in the morning for special situations where maximum cognitive function is required. While Huperzine A appears to be safe for special situations, daily use could remotely lead to undesirable complications such as acetylcholine accumulation. Therefore, it should not be taken more than a few times a week at the most. If taken more often, "acetylcholine overload" could result. These are usually minor (muscle tension, headaches) and can easily be avoided by reducing the dose. In a double-blind Chinese study of the effect of Huperzine on Alzheimer's patients, 50 patients were given daily dosages for eight weeks, and 53 subjects were given placebo. Nearly 60 percent of the patients on Huperzine improved. "No severe side effect was found." Huperzine A is available in 50 mcg size in some health food stores and by mail from Life Extension, 1/800/877-2447).

## $$$$ Indole-3-Carbinol

Indole-3-Carbinol frequently referred to as 13C is an anti-estrogen similar to Tamoxifen, the approved therapy for breast cancer, but working a bit differently. This compound is naturally found in cruciferous vegetables (brussel sprouts, broccoli , and cauliflower). Specifically 13C alters the way estrogen is metabolized in the body from the "bad" to the "good" pathway greatly reducing 16 alpha hydroxylations. This bad metabolite similar to most pesticides is a tumor promoter. 13C prevents a buildup of these xenoestrogens from the body. Additionally, 13C boosts the immune function by T-cell enhancement. This naturally occurring phytonutrient has no down side, costing about $40 for a month's supply of 250 mg. capsules twice a day. These can be ordered from Vitamins Research, 1/800/877-2447.

### $$$$ Inositol Hexaphosphate (IP$_6$)

IP$_6$, also in the past, was called InsP$_6$ and phytic acid. Inositol is a B vitamin and its derivative, IP$_6$ is a natural component of some grain and legumes, particularly soybeans. Thanks go to A.M. Shansudden, M.D., PhD., a professor of Pathology at the University of Maryland School of Medicine, who has spent the last 15 years identifying and researching this fantastic compound. Although used primarily by the community of alternative medical doctors and some clever practicing orthodox oncologist (medical cancer doctors), in that it suppresses almost all types of cancer, but it has some other fantastic benefits for longevity.

IP$_6$ has many actions conducive to longevity. It is a premier antioxidant. Independently, it regulates the oxygen compassity of our red blood cells. Moreover, IP$_6$ reduces both cholesterol and trigylceride, as well as preventing heart damage during a heart attack. In diabetes, it not only improves insulin sensitivity, but decreases its complications. In addition to the above, prevention of the most common type of kidney stone (calcium oxibate) is suppressed by IP$_6$. In preliminary studies, it prevents depression and may work adjunctively in schizophrenia. The all important function of enhancing of our immune system, by increasing the activity of our natural killer (NK) cells, may make IP$_6$ a preventative to infection and cancer.

IP$_6$ is as safe as water. We naturally can increase our

intake by consuming the outer layer of grains (rice, wheat, rye), but soybean seed is the best source with its whole seed (bean) containing up to 26% of IP6. I recommend 1-2 grams a day, taken between meals twice a day to avoid its interaction with protein in the diet. For individuals with a high risk of cancer, cardiovascular disease, kidney stone, etc., 2-4 grams a day. Finally, to help existing cancer, 5-8 grams a day. The product is available without prescription in most health food stores. It is supplied in 500 mg (1/2 gram) capsules and is made by several manufacturers. The best and the one who has participated in much of its research is Enzymatic Therapy (800-783-2286) in Greenbay, WI.

### $$ Lactoferrin (See page 202)

### $$$ Lipoic Acid

Perhaps the most important substance that has been variously called "the universal antioxidant" or the "ideal oxidant" is lipoic acid, sometimes called thiotic acid. You can think of lipoic acid as a kind of "wild card" antioxidant. Evidence shows that even if you are not getting enough vitamin C or E, for example, lipoic acid supplements can make up at least part of the deficit. Recent studies have demonstrated that lipoic acid stops cholesterol uptake by the vessel wall, intracellular damage by free radicals, discourage the formation of damaging molecules, growth of cancer cells, and possibly even improve memory. In addition to being a powerful antioxidant, lipoic acid has an important role in controlling blood sugar. Through both of these mechanisms, it may help prevent the negative effects of having an even slightly elevated blood sugar causing some of the serious side effects of diabetes (nerve damage, pain, blindness, heart disease and accelerated aging). It may even help repair some of the nerve damage that may have occurred by encouraging new nerve growth.

Lipoic acid is also a super-chelator, capable of removing form our bodies excess iron, calcium, copper, toxic molecules such as cadmium, lead and mercury, as well as organic hydrocarbons. Lipoic acid is considered a conditionally vital antioxidant nutrient. Specifically, the body makes some of its own lipoic acid, but we still need to get most of it from external sources, either from food, such as meat, or supplements. Our ability to make lipoic acid does decline with age. In addition to its ability it scavenges free radicals on its own Lipoic acid also enhances the actions of many other antioxidants such as glutathione and vitamin E. It can either substitute for them when they are deficient, or help to recycle them after they have neutralized free radical molecules. An excess fasting blood sugar greater than 110 or 140 after eating, cause glycation of living tissue, which is liken to our tissues "rusting" and not working too well in this state (see page 214). The blood sugar reacts spontaneously and directly with proteins such as collagen (found in skin, blood vessels, connective tissue and nerves). Over the years, glycation does accelerate tissue aging and promotes kidney damage, atherosclerosis and loss of vision, all of which are common diabetic complications as well as noted in just aging. Lipoic acid, like insulin, reduces glycation, enhancing the movement of blood sugar into our cells. It promotes greater energy production by muscles and reduces the amount of glucose stored as fat. It is not the cholesterol per se, but the oxidized cholesterol that is preferentially taken up by the white cells within the artery wall. So when LDL cholesterol is changed by oxidation or free radicals, this begins a process that ends up with the formation of fatty deposits on the inner walls of arteries, reduced blood flow, heart attacks and strokes!!

Antioxidants, like vitamin E, protect LDL from oxidation and free radicals. However, in the process of LDL, vitamin E itself is consumed. Lipoic acid helps recycle vitamin E molecules, so they join the battle again and again. Additionally, lipoic acid itself provides antioxidant protections from LDL. A colleague of mine, Dr. Richard Passwater, has shown that lipoic acid may reduce blood cholesterol by 40 percent and LDL levels by 42 percent in lab animals. Lipoic acid is safe with no side effects. In over three decades of use in Europe, no study has shown any serious adverse effects of taking lipoic acid supplements. The recommended "therapeutic dose" for healthy adults is 100-200mg. By contrast, animal studies have shown the acute toxic dose to be ten times that of the therapeutic dose. There is no interference with any other drug I know of. It may be taken once a day with any supplement or food. It is supplied in 25, 50, 100, and 200mg capsules.

## $$ Lutein

Lutein protects and perhaps improves the outlook on cancer of the colon and macular degeneration (see page 118). It seems to protect the sporadic colonic cancer rather than the familial type (American Journal of Clinical Nutrition; 2000: Feb; 71(2);575-82. It is an effective antioxidant in the body and is found in the region of the retina called the macula and in the lens of the eye. The macula is an area of the central retina responsible for clear reading and color vision. Lutein and its isomer zeaxanthin are the only two carotenoids found in the eye. Other carotenoids like, beta-carotene, and vitamin A are not found in the eye and are not associated with reducing age-related macular degeneration. Zeaxanthin is generally less available and the dose is 264 mg a day. Naturally, Lutein is found in dark green vegetable leaves, spinach being the food with one of the highest amounts per serving.

Macular degeneration is a retinal disorder that obscures central vision among an estimated 4 million Americans and is the leading cause of blindness in people over age 60. Persons with macular degeneration often have lower levels of Lutein and zeaxanthin in the macula. Zinc (see page 182) is also used in conjunction with Lutein. Currently, there are no effective treatments for macular degeneration and, therefore, ways to reduce the prevalence of the disease is critical, including the addition of Lutein to the diet or as a supplement. In addition, there is evidence indicating that Lutein and zeaxanthin reduce cataract formation.

## $$$ Lycopene

Lycopene is one of the 600 plus carotenoids known to man. Unlike most of the others, carotenoids, man does not metabolize it to vitamin A. Lycopene provides stronger antioxidant protection against certain types of free radicals, and may protect against particular cancers better than any nutrient presently known. Lycopene makes up about half the carotenes in human blood.

Lycopene is what gives tomatoes, watermelons, grapefruits and papaya their red color. A pigment synthesized by some plants and animals to protect them from the sun, lycopene evolved as a weapon against certain types of free radicals. Lycopene is more effective at quenching free radicals, then vitamin E in one study on oxidized fat.

Recently reported in the journal *Lipids*, a group from Canada demonstrated that lycopene significantly lowers LDL oxidation in human blood. What's interesting is that lycopene works better in combination with lutein, another carotenoid which is found in spinach (see page 233). Lutein is associated with maintenance of the macula. People with high cholesterol have been found to have high levels of free radicals and low levels of lycopene and beta carotene.

Humans get most of their lycopene from tomatoes, by far the richest source. Tomato products offer a more concentrated source of lycopene than the fresh fruit itself. For example, tomato powder contains approximately 120 mg per 100 grams of fruit, whereas fresh tomatoes have only 2 mg per 100. Since lycopene is a nutrient that can stand the heat, cooked tomato products, such as tomato paste, provide more of it than fresh tomatoes. Spaghetti sauce is an adequate source of lycopene because it contains fat, which is necessary for absorption. It has been theorzed that heating tomatoes makes their lycopene more absorbable.

Just as lutein is concentrated in the macula, lycopene is concentrated in the prostate gland. Researchers at the University of Bern report that lycopene added to prostate cancer cells in the test tube, and the addition of other cofactors markedly reduced the cancer cell growth. Lycopene by itself doesn't work. Several studies have linked lycopene with a lower risk of prostate cancer. One of these studies, the Washington County study, found that men with the most lycopene in their blood halved their risk of prostate cancer compared to those with the least. For those under 70 years old, the benefit of tomato products and found lower risk with higher consumption. Tomato sauce, as opposed to juice which had no effect.

Several studies show a connection between lycopene and cancer prevention. Lycopene appears to be protective against cancer of the digestive tract. Several studies have found a lower risk for colorectal cancer in people who eat a lot of tomato products and/or have higher levels of lycopene in their blood. More direct evidence has been provided by researchers in Japan who did a study on colon cancer in rats. They found that tomato juice provided significant protection against a chemical carcinogen (N-methylnitrosourea). It's important to note, however, that pure lycopene did not. The authors of the study speculate that lycopene's action depends on other factors present in the juice that is missing in pure lycopene. Recent thinking in carotene research is that the carotenes are both interdependent and dependent on other vitamins and minerals, and this must be taken into account when studying them. Another cancer that mayt relate to lycopene is pancreatic. Researchers at Johns Hopkins tested the stored blood for 22 people with pancreatic cancer, for levels of certain vitamins and selenium. (Blood was drawn before treatment). Lycopene and selenium levels were lower in patients than controls. The dose of lycopene is 10 and 15 mg capsules, twice a day. There seems to be no side effects.

## $ Melatonin

Melatonin comes form the remnant of the body of our third eye. This, our pineal gland, contains light sensitive cells and monitors our environment. It keeps our body in tune with the daily and seasonal change. Hence, we are synchronous with nature; rest and sleep when it is dark and active and awake when it is light; and in lower animal, the sense of when to migrate, mate and hibernate. Melatonin is 10 to 20 times higher at night than during the day and is one to two times higher on June 21 than on December 21 Melatonin is passed through the placenta before birth, in mother's milk in the early part of our lives and gradually increases until age seven, when it greatly increases. At puberty, there is a temporary decline, which signals the pituitary to release the sex stimulating hormones. At about the age of 40, our pineal gland shrinks and later becomes calcified. By age 60, our melatonin production is half of what it was at age 20. In addition to extending our youthful life, melatonin restores normal sleep patterns, is an antioxidant, strengthens our immune system and enhances sexual vitality, as well as preventing jet lag. It is non addictive and, if taken in the proper dosage, *does not have any downside* except its expense and in minority of people, vivid dreams. I recommend 3 to 9 mg one hour before desired sleep (3mg at ages 30 to 40; 6mg at ages 40 to 60; and 9mg after age 60). It is also available in sublingual (under the tongue) tablets, in which case it is 2.5mg from ages 30 to 40; 5mg from ages 40 to 60; and 7.5mg after age 60. The pills come in varying sizes, which include a 3mg oral preparation and a 2.5mg and 5mg under the tongue product.

### $$$$ MGN-3

This is a natural immune complex derived from a mushroom and is said to triple natural killer (NK) cell function. The natural killer cells help rid our body of foreign substances, such as cancer cells and bacteria. The B and T cells are white cells (lymphocytes) that produce chemicals that attack foreign substance. Hopefully this happens before the substances do us harm. It provides more NK-cell efficacy than most advanced mushroom extract, vitamin or herbal products according to the manufacturer. *It can be used adjunctively or alone in various cancers, Hepatitis C, chronic fatigue syndrome (see page 253). It should, with other supplements or a "stand alone drug," increase our longevity by delaying or preventing disease. MGN-3 (Arabinoxylane Compound – Patent #5560914) enzymatically integrates rice bran with medicinal mushroom extract via hydrolysis. This combination improves systemic absorption, increasing the effect of MGN-3's immunity-enhancing properties;

There are virtually no side effects. It is supplied in 250 mg capsules of which one, three times a day is recommended. For information call LaneLabs at 800-526-3005.

## $$ MSM

MSM (Methyl Sulfonyl Methane) is an odorless, tasteless breakdown product of DMSO. It provides a sulfur foundation that the body needs to form proteins, collagen synthesis, activate vitamins and maintain the immune system. It has also been shown to grow thick hair, strong nails and improve the skin texture. MSM relieves swelling, inflammation and pain because it more easily allows the harmful substances that have accumulated to flow out and nutrients to flow in. It contributes sulfur to the body needed to make vitamins such as $B_1$ and the antioxidant aminoacid glutathione. MSM helps the liver excrete toxins. Additionally, it provides structure to the glucosamine needed for healthy ligaments, tendons, heart valves, etc. It is without any side effects. People can take as many as 100 grams of this without ill effect. I would suggest starting with 2 grams (2000 milligrams) and every week, increase by 1000 milligrams to a total of 8 grams. It can be taken with or without food. It is available in capsules, dissolvable crystals and powder. The powder is usually put in juice, and some mix it with food such as applesauce or oatmeal and has absolutely no taste. The price of MSM is relatively inexpensive, costing about $10.00 for sixty 1000 milligram capsules. MSM is "safe as water" and "cheap as dirt"! It can be purchased in bulk for much less. One can buy this for under $12.40 a pound and divide it up accordingly. You can contact a veterinary supply company, Jeffers, at 1-800-JEFFERSS, or a 24-hour fax, 417-256-1550, or write to P.O. Box 948, West Plains, Missouri 65775-0948. One teaspoon is 4 grams.

## $ N-Acetyl Cysteine

The oral cysteine that is best tolerated is called N-Acetyl Cysteine (NAC). Cysteine is the rate limiting amino acid in the production of glutathione. By that I mean that if you are low in cysteine, the production of glutathione can not move forward. Many studies have shown that supplementtion of cysteine has led to increased intercellular levels of glutathione. The food that contains most cysteine is egg yolk. Although eaten two or three times a week should cause no problems with ones cholesterol, the problem is that cysteine may bypass the glutathione pathway and go to a useless amino acid cysteine. The same is true with tking the plain amino acid L-Cystine. Glutamine supplementation aids in the production of Glutathione. However, L-Cysteine itself is poorly tolerated and is quickly changed to the amino acid cystine.

Therefore, it is best to take N-Acetyl Cysteine which is better tolerated, better absorbed and is used to make glutathione. Usually people tolerate up to 2g daily without problems.

### $$$$ Noni Juice

Noni juice or sometimes referred to as Tahitian noni juice is the liquid extract of the Polynesian plant, *Morinde citifolian*. Reputedly, the plant has been used for centuries, both internally and externally, by the Polynesians for its healing properties. A consortium bought up all the rights to process and sell the product. In the U.S., it is distributed by multilevel marketing. Among the other phytochemicals, it contains G-D-glucopyranose pentaacetab, which enhance the cytokine from the macrophages of our immune system. This helps not only to fight infection, but to ward off cancer. Additionally, the plant has several constitutients that improve tissue growth. Another of its chemicals is Damnacanthal that reverses the chromosomal makeup of a cancer cell towards a normal architecture. Other properties increase one's stamina, improve bowel function, and makes weight loss easier. Although there is some scientific proof for these claims, I feel the product is more hype than fact. It can be obtained from over 15,000 distributions in the U.S. alone.

## $$$$ Oxitriptan

Oxitriptan is converted into the brain hormone, serotonin in the body. Serotonin is a key factor in mood regulation, eating disorders, and anxiety. Serotonin is also the precursor to the pineal gland's production of melatonin. Oxitriptan's anti-aging benefits may include the prevention and treatment of depression, maintenance of serotonin levels as the body ages, prevention and treatment of compulsive disorders like overeating, improved daytime alertness and treatment of insomnia. Side effects include nausea and mild gastric discomfort. Oxitriptan is supplied in 50mg or 100mg tablets under the trade names Cincofarm, Levotonine, Levothym, Oxyfan, Serotonyl™, Serovit, Telesol, Trimag, Tript-OG, Tript-Oh, Triptenetm and Triptum™.

## $$$$ Piracetam

The world's best-selling nootropic (brain nourisher) drug, piracetam, is purported to prevent and correct memory loss due to old age, sharpening memory and improving clarity and attention to detail. It brings about important metabolic modifications in nerve cells, which results in greater receptiveness and increased use of chemical energy. Piracetam's anti-aging benefits include treatment and prevention of age-related mental decline, protection of the brain against aging damage and environmental toxins, increased potential life span, improved alertness, awareness and short- to medium-term memory. Side effects may include nausea, dizziness and headaches. Patients with renal disorders should use piracetam with caution.

Piracetam is available by presscription at certain pharmacies in 400mg, 600mg, 800mg, and 1200mg tablets, and in an oral liquid form. Trade name preparations include Avigilen, Axonyl, Braintop, Cerebrofortem, Cerebropan, Cerebrosteriltm, Cerebryl, Cerepar N, Cetam, Ciclofalina, Cuxabraintam, Encetrop, Flavis, Gabacet, Genogris, Geram, Geratam, Memo Puretam, Noodis, Nootrop, Nootropyl, Normabrain, Norzetam, Novocetam, Pirabene, Piracebraltam, Piracetrop, Psycoton and Sinapsan.

While some of the generic forms of piracetam may be acceptable, generic piracetam may be a "hit or miss" affair. There are now a growing number of piracetam look alikes, including Oxiracetam, Aniracetam, Modiracetam, and Pramiracetam. Oxiracetam is the industry standard in Europe and when new analogues are developed they are compared to Oxiracetam.

### $$$ Phosphatidylserine (PS)

Phosphatidylserine (PS) is a naturally occurring phospholipid, essential for the membranes of all cells, particularly in the brain. Hence it is another smart drug. Taken at night this substance gives a good sleep. It has some promising effects in stress related brain decline that take its toll over the decades. Stress causes the pituatary gland to secrete an adrenal cortisol stimulator, ACTH. Two recent studies from Italy have shown that PS is able to blunt the ACTH and cortisol response to stressors. This means that individuals whose pituitary adrenal drive is overstimulated may be able to take oral PS to reduce this bad response to stress. Researchers found that in just 10 days, a dose of 800mg/day was sufficient to drop both ACTH and cortisol under the stressors that would otherwise induce significant increases of both. PS has been effective in Alzheimer's disease and does improve both remote and recent momory of normals. It may forstall or prevent Alzheimer's that will occur in every one of us if we live long enough. In some, it may not occur until we are 140!

### $$ Pregnenolone

Pregnenolone is the basic material of all human steroid manufacture, including DHEA, progesterone, testosterone and estrogen. It blocks the effects of cortisol, preventing and stimulates brain NMDA receptors. These receptors, which decline with age, play a role in the function of synapses and neurons, influencing learning, memory, and cognitive function. Pregnenolone's anti-aging benefits include reduction of stress, reduction of arthritic inflammation, potential maintenance of memory capability, improved mood, well-being, and the ability to see and smell better. There are no side effects. It is supplied in 5mg, 10mg, 20mg, 25mg, 30mg, 50mg and 100mg capsules without a prescription. I recommend 20 to 30 mg a day.

## $ Primrose

Known botanically as *Oenothera biennis*, oil of evening primrose (OEP) is used by women to help relieve breast pain and symptoms of the premenstrual syndrome. OEP is also believed by some to decrease the risk of other conditions, such as cardiovascular disease and rheumatoid arthritis. The effects of OEP are attributed to its high concentrations of the fatty acids cis-linoleic acid and cis-y-linolenic acid (GLA). Both are produced in the body in limited amounts. Women with breast pain have reduced levels of GLA. Supplementation of 2.4 to 3.2 g/d of OEP (in divided doses) has been shown to decrease pain in 44% of women with cyclical breast pain and 50% of those with noncyclical breast pain such as with hormone replacement. OEP must be taken for at least four months before its effects will be felt. OEP can also be used topically.

Women with PMS are also believed to have decreased conversion of cis-linoleic acid to GLA. The resulting reduction in GLA levels leads to deficient synthesis of prostaglandin E1, which is thought to aggravate PMS Symptoms. In one study, administration of 4 capsules of OEP (each containing 72% linoleic acid and 9% GLA) twice daily during the last 14 days of the menstrual cycle relieved PMS symptoms. However, conclusive results concerning the effectiveness of OEP for PMS are lacking, because other studies have shown no effect.

OEP is relatively free of side effects, although mild gastrointestinal irritation has been reported. OEP has no known drug interactions. Most studies evaluating the use of OEP have used products containing 72% cislinoleic acid and 9% GLA. Patients should use a brand of OEP that contain these amounts of fatty acids, and they should follow the manufacturer's guidelines for dosing.

## $ Procaine

Procaine, a local anathestic, was first used to reverse aging in modern times by the Romanian physician, Anna Aslan. She suggested in 1956 that procaine was helpful to combat arthritis, arteriosclerosis, senile skin changes, baldness and aging in general. Procaine improves the metabolism of fat, enhancing its bodily distribution. It increases the rate of excretion of certain harmful hormones (ketosteroids), which usually increases with age. It improves a sense of well-being and perhaps increased potential life span. Side effects are only allergic reactions. Procaine can be administered by injection or by tablet. Procaine is available in 50mg or 100mg tablets under the names GH-3 and KH-3 orally and by prescription for the injectable variety. It is frequently used in the solution for chelation therapy.

## $$$ Progesterone

Progesterone is also produced by the ovaries and compliments estrogen. Natural progesterone has far less side effects than the synthetic varieties, called progestins such as methylprogesterone (Provera). However, the micronized progesterone, Prometrium® works as well is, however, more costly. Specifically, unopposed estrogens cause mood swings, fluid retention, migraine headaches and a decrease in life expectancy. Progesterone by prescription is available as a topical, oral or a sublingual preparation. Also there are several excellent topical products such as Projest™. (See Chapter Eight.)

## $$$ Prolotherapy

Prolotherapy is not a supplement, but a treatment to strengthen the ligaments and tendons by proliferation of new cells. Similar to a rubberband, a ligament or tendon can become "over stretched." The resulting laxity can cause pain as cartilage rub together or muscles are over-worked as they tighten in an attempt to stabilize the bones. According to some experts, this is actually the cause of most osteoarthritis. It is used for myofascial syndromes. A proliferative solution such as concentrated glucose is injected directly into the site of the weakened ligament. The body's own immune system grows new and healthy tissue which stabilizes the bones and joints, relieving musculoskeletal pain. Prolotherapy is used to rejuvenate specific parts of our aging body. Unfortunately, it is performed by only a handful of physicians in this country.

## $$ Propolis

Propolis is a resin obtained from the buds of some trees and flowers. This sap is rich in such nutrients as minerals and the B vitamins. Bees collect it along with pollen. Propolis is through to contain a natural antibiotic, called galangin, and is used in a variety of remedies to treat or prevent low-grade infections, especially in people who do not want to take antibiotics. Bees spread the propolis around their hives to protect them from bacteria and viruses. The name "propolis" comes from Greek words meaning "defenses before a town." Reputedly, propolis improves energy and endurance and helps immunity by stimulating thymus activity. It is available from bee keepers or at health food stores.

## Pyruvate

According to the human studies, Pyruvate improves exercise performance by enhancing the transport of glucose into the muscle cell. This chemical, a natural antioxidant, occurs naturally in the body and is an end product of the metabolism of sugar or starch shifting the kreb cycle into fat burning. A paper presented in *The Proceeding of the Society for Experimental Biology and Medicine* in spring of 2000 detailed that Pyruvate forms the high energy bond ATP. This increased the mechanical performance of the heart, particularly when injured by decreased blood flow. Therefore Pyruvate is very helpful for heart failure and as a weight loss aid. Being extremely safe, it can be bought in health food stores in 1 gram capsules. The recommended dosage is 1 capsule 30 minutes before meals.

## $ Pycnogenol

Pycnogenol benefits-20 to 30 times more potent antioxidant than vitamin C or E. It is particularly good for free radical protection in cells with limited blood flow, such as linings of inflamed joints, elastin and neurons.

## Red Yeast Rice

Red yeast rice, which is the generic form of Cholestin, can be purchased relatively inexpensively with forty-five 600 mg capsules costing about $12. The dose is two capsules with supper. This comes from the yeast strain *Monachus purpureus,* which is the fermentation of rice. The compound contains 3% Lovastatin (Mevacor). The FDA is trying to make this a drug rather than an over-the-counter product. It can lower the choelsterol 12-15% and is extremely safe. Taking grapefruit and/or the inexpensive antibiotic, erythromycin with it with an 18% reduction makes the combination even more potent.

## $$$$ RN13

RN13 acts on cell respiration and metabolism in most of our organs to include our brain. It contains 13 different animal source RNAs, as well as vitamins, amino acids, procaine and glutamic acid and biolecithin. RNA is responsible for protein biosynthesis and helps repair and regenerate our tissues. The animal source RNAs from specific organs may stimulate the same organs in humans. RN13 has been shown to make aging individuals more alert and vital and to improve weak concentration, defective memory, anxiety, troubled sleep and lack of appetite.

RN13 is a multi combination product, of which each liquid capsule contains macromolecular organ substances out of embryo 0.37ng, placenta 0.1ng, amnion 6-pg, funiculus umbilical 60pg, cor 0.2ng, pancreas 0.1ng, mucosa intest 0.1ng, glandular suprarenal 0.lng, glandular parathyroid 20pg, testes juv. And fet. 0.2ng; as well as mixture of the following drug additives; heparin 5x10-3 IU, L-glutamic acid 10ug, methenolone acetate 4ng, trijod thyroxin HCl 4pg, vitamin E 40ng, vitamin B12 40ng, vitamin B6 40ng, p-amino benzoyldiethylaminoethanol HCL (Procaine) 8ng, biolecithin 10mg, trace elements (Fe, Co, Cu, Mg, Zn, Ca) 1.5ng, sodium dodecyl sulfate 15ug, medium chained triglyceride 410mg.

Side effects are rare but may include mild irritation at the site of an injection and minor allergic reactions such as a skin rash. People suffering disturbances in purine metabolism, such as gout, should avoid RN13 therapy. Antibiotics and drugs that suppress the immune system may inhibit RN13's efficacy. RN13 is administered by injection and supplemented by ampules or capsules. In less severe cases 2ml ampules and 0.5ml liquid capsules are available. VitOrgan of Germany manufactures RN13 under the trade name NeyGeront.

## $$ Royal Jelly

Royal jelly is another panacea for health and longevity seekers. Worker bees make this exotic substance for their queen bee who grows initially five times faster and eight times as large as the worker bee. Royal jelly is an energizer. It is high in certain unique fatty acids, simple carbohydrates, and pantothenic acid, which is supportive of the adrenals. It also contains the other B vitamins, all of the essential amino acids, and many minerals, such as iron, calcium, silicon, sulfur, and potassium. Royal jelly has been used to support weight loss, as it is a rich and energizing nutrient yet low in calories (20 calories per teaspoon), and to treat problems such as fatigue, insomnia, digestive disorders, ulcers, and cardiovascular ailments. But many people, especially women, experience an uplifting feeling when they take the semi-solid liquid or encapsulated royal jelly. It is available in all health food stores and from beekeepers.

## $$$$ S-Adenosylmethionine (SAMe)

The price was prohibitive up to two years of age. Thanks to competition which "makes the world go round," the price of this very useful compound is within most of our grasps. This one pill has many uses. Although it's used for liver disease in Russia, arthritis in Germany and depression in Italy, it is used in this country for fibromyalgia and chronic fatigue. In dozens of European trials involving thousands of patients over decades, this product has had a sterling record. It is an approved drug in fourteen countries. In many of these countries, such as Germany, it is paid for by insurance.

SAMe, formally known as S-adenosylmethionine is not a herb or hormone. It is a molecule that all living cells, including our own, produce constantly. It is involved in the all-important chemical reaction that is seen not only in higher living forms, but also many lower ones called METHYLATION. According to some researchers, methylation occurs a billion times a second throughout the body and affects everything from fetal development to brain function. It actually regulates the expression of genes. It does this by its action on various hormones and neurotransmitters. Serotonin, adrenalin, melatonin and dopamine are but a few of these substances that are produced because of SAMe and its effect on methylation. In a trial involving 22,000 patients, SAMe was as effective as NSAID's such as ibuprofen, and Nalfon, but unlike these, instead of speeding the breakdown of cartilage, it helps to restore this and indeed may be preventative in the development of degenerative arthritis that most of us will get as we become older. In a study done at a California medical school, using doses as high as 1600 mg a day, a few percent of patients had an upset stomach and a rare patient, who were treated with the newer antidepressants called SSRI's (Prozac, Zoloft, etc.), became manic. SAMe does not interact adversely with any other medications. It has helped two-thirds of my patients with chronic fatigue syndrome and fibromyalgia over the two years I have used it.

The usual dose of this is taken on an empty stomach, 200 mg twice a day. The vitamin company, Pharmavite, has a brand called "Nature Made," which costs $35 for fifty. This is foil-covered and enteric coated. As a methyldoner, it reduces homocysteine which is probably more important in producing hardening of the arteries, then even cholesterol, and hence reduces strokes and heart attacks.

## $ Sea Cucumber

The Chinese have relied on this maritime medicinal creature for thousands of years. Australians named it an official arthritis drug fifteen years ago. Sea cucumber products come with the ground animal parts at a dose of one to two grams a day. Also it is available with several other products to include sea plants, glucosamine (see page 227) and activated fatty acids (see page 226). Although some physicians feel this is a wonderful adjunct for arthritis care, my experience in a handful of patients indicate this to be only moderately effective. It is very safe and not too expensive.

## $$$ Testosterone

Androgens (testosterone) in small amounts is made in the woman's ovary and adrenal gland, as well as the testes in males. For men around the age of 40, testosterone begins to drop. For women, it wanes after 50. This is accompanied by a decrease in libido, difficulty in erectile function, lethargy, weight gain, loss of muscle and bone mass. I test testosterone levels, and if less than 800 for men, consider prescribing this very important hormone. As a prescription, it is available as a patch, lotion, a pill, and as an injection. For women, testosterone in a smaller dose is usually added to the estrogen (Estratest™) or in a combination with estrogen and progesterone by a compounding pharmacy. Not only does the testosterone cause improvement of hot flashes in women, but enhances the effects of Viagra™ in men. I have recommended this applied vaginally to help orgasm in women.

## $ Thyroid Hormone

Thyroid hormone is not for everyone, although it does naturally decline with age or stress. Clinically, I routinely check a TSH (Thyroid Stimulating Hormone) level, which is a pituitary hormone. Paradoxically, the higher this level is, the lower output our thyroid has. So, if the TSH is greater than 5, it indicates deficiency in thyroid output and/or production. Some doctors measure the actual hormone (T3 and/or T4), but the TSH is a more accurate biosensitive marker for thyroid activity. Low thyroid activity causes fatigue, weight gain, decreases hearing, dry skin, thinning of the hair, lowering of the voice and premature aging.

Body temperature is regulated by thyroid function. Holistic physicians advocate taking the temperature to diagnose hypothyroidism (low thyroid) by a glass oral thermometer. Taken every three hours, starting three hours after getting up, three times, for three days. The further the temperature is lowered from 98.6 degrees, the more likely we are to have a functional (E. Dennis Wilson Syndrome, page 283) or anatomic hypothyroidism.

Heart rate is also decreased with lower thyroid, but there are many other factors such as medication, heart disease and being "over athletic" which can also cause low heart rate and I don't recommend this to diagnose low thyroid. If one suspects hyperthyroid, one should then get the TSH level to document this abnormal state, since taking excess or not need thyroid hormones could cause osteoporosis.

Thyroid hormone is a prescription drug and is supplied by drops, pills or capsules but is usually taken orally. The synthetic version is recommended by most traditional physicians. Recently, the generic brand has been proven to be as effective as the brand names, such as Synthroid™. I usually recommend the natural thyroid. Used for a hundred years, this was abandoned. Although obtained from cattle, there is no need to worry about mad cow disease. Natural thyroid has a combination of T4, T3, T2, T 1. The synthetic (Synthroid™) thyroid produced by the drug companies uses only the T4 and rarely only T3 (Cytomel™). The active molecule is converted from the T4 to the active T3 and occasionally the inactive form called Reverse T3 is produced. Additionally, the T1 and T2 have some role in thyroid function, although scientifically it is not well worked out. Also, there may be some chaperone molecules in the natural product, ushering the thyroid better into the cells. Natural is much more forgiving than using the synthetic thyroid. The dose is between 30 and 365 mg a day and should not be taken with calcium supplements.

If one takes thyroid, a repeat TSH should be done in three to six weeks and if this level is still high, a higher dose of thyroid is prescribed. Repeat studies are done until the TSH is less than 5. In general, the higher the TSH, the more thyroid is recommended. An ill or older patient should gradually increase his dosage until the desired amount has been established. Twice yearly, the TSH should be repeated. Two blood tests can be affected by consumption of this hormone. It can influence the protime in patients in common consistently taking Coumadin (Warfarin). Also, it will lower the cholesterol and tryglycerides in most individuals. Side effects are that of excess thyroid (hyperthroidism) includes nervousness, weight loss, sweats, decrease tolerance to heat, rapid heart action and insomnia.

### $$$ Thym-Uvocal

Thym-Uvocal contains a standardized combination of thymus peptides, which replaces the decrease of thymic secretion associated with increasing age. The thymic secretion influences our immune system It appears to have a favorable action on the T-4/T-8 cell ratio, and thus a stimulating and modulating action on the cellular immune system. ThymUvocal increases levels of antibodies and phagocytosis, increases interleukin-1 production, and activates macrophages and enhances their tumor cell destruction action.

It is also used in the treatment of infection , cancer, rheumatic disease, and dermatology disorders. The latter includes matitis and psoriasis. It contains protein-free dry substances from calf thymus extract. There is a possibility of allergic minor reactions as a side effect. Thym-Uvocal is available in 2ml ampules, topical cream and 240mg tablets. Mulli of Germany manufactures it.

## $$$$ Thymic Protein

Thymic protein is a generic form of the above and works similarly. The standard dosage for healthy people is 2 micrograms per day.

## $$ Trimethylglycine (TMG)

In the past called Betaine, trimethylglycine is a methyl donor supplement that helps protect cellular DNA from mutation. As humans age, methyl groups do decrease. It does lower homocysteine with and without vitamins B12, B6 and folic acid. Please see the discussion of homocysteine in other places in this book.

TMG is in a powdered form from Klabin Marketing, and is found in many over the counter preparations in health food stores. An inexpensive variety is with Betaine HCL used to produce stomach acid. It is not as potent a methyl doner as SAMe (page 245), but is much less expensive

## $$$$ Vasopressin

Vasopressin is a hormone secreted by the posterior portion of the pituitary gland. While it legitimately used to prevent frequent urination, in bed wetting patterns. It is used to treat memory deficits due to old age (senile dementia), drug toxicity and amnesia. Whenever a memory is deposited in the brain, vasopressin regulates the process. Vasopressin benefits one by enhanced clarity, increased attention to detail, and improved short and long term memory. It has been shown to actually raise the IQ.

Side effects are minimal. There is occasional nasal itchiness, and rarely headaches, conjunctivitis, sore throat, nausea, abdominal pain and the urgent need to defecate as a result of increased bowel stimulation. It should be administered with caution of hypertension, epilepsy, arteriosclerosis. Vasopressin is available in 5ml or 12m1 nasal sprays under the trade names Diapid, Lypressin Injection BP 1993, Lypressin Nasal Solution USP 23, Neo-Lidocatonr™, Postacton, Postacton™, Syntopressin, Vasopresina, Vasopressin, Vasopressin™, Vasopressine, and Vasopressine™.

### $$$ Vinpocetine

Vinpocetine (vin-paw-seh-teen) improves brain energy and blood supply and has been used as a preventative and a treatment of stroke injury. It acts as a cerebral metabolic activator, which may improve cerebral circulation and enhance oxygen and glucose utilization in the brain as it is a cognitive enhancer, sharpening mental alertness and memory. Vinpocetine may diminish brain dysfunction due to hypoxia or poor cerebral metabolism. It improves oxygen and glucose utilization by brain cells and increase their resistance to damage by poor circulation. It improves eyesight, hearing, and concentration Side effects are very rare, but may include nausea. It too is a smart drug.

This is an extract of Vinca minor (periwinkle). Vinpocetine is supplied in 1mg, 5mg and 10mg tablets under the trade names Cavinton™, Remedial™, and Vincaton™. Thirty to forty mg a day are recommended. There are no interactions with other drugs and virtually no side effects.

*"When health is absent, wisdom cannot reveal itself, art cannot become manifest, strength cannot be exerted, wealth becomes useless and reason is powerless."*
*Herophilus, circa 300 BC*

## Figure 5-I

## Conflict

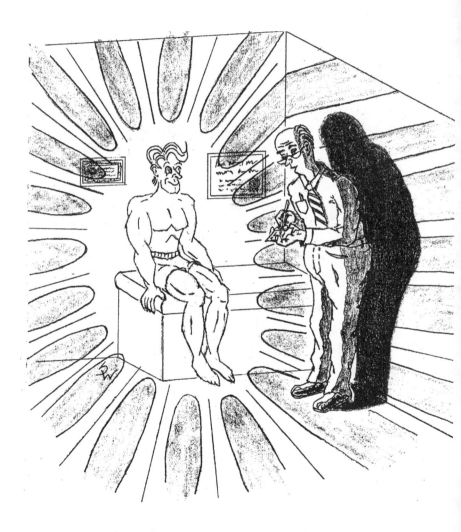

"Steve, you are almost 100 years old and should know better. Those vitamins and supplements won't help. Here, take this prescription."

# SIX

# The F Word

Chronic Fatigue Syndrome and its sister, Fibromyalgia Syndrome are in everyone's vocabulary, although as common Myofascial Syndrome is not. The F letter hence is in the initials CFS, FMS, and MFS. Myalgic encephalomyelitis may be the scientific term for this collection of symptoms. This does have a "F" in it, although spelled "ph'. Is F indicative of *fatigue, fascial,* and *fibromyalgia,* or is it for the foreboding, fearful, freaky, fickle, flighty fault of human nature? The fitful, feverfish, fainty, foul, forgetful symptoms may indicate the fermentation of this fungating disease that is now a fashionable foe in our society. Perhaps the F word would be a better term for this fretful, formidable, futile, frightening and at times, furious problem. Muscle fatigue and pain affects nearly 50 percent of any patient who seeks medical care. Fatigue also is common in many of the diseases that range from not enough sleep to something more serious, such as depression, infection, or the worst, cancer! A critical life event, either physical or mental frequently precedes most patients with the F Syndrome. In general, the diagnosis of F Syndrome is usually made by excluding other identifiable diseases, such as infectious, psychiatric or specific environmental causes. The incidence of this set of diseases, in which 9 million in the United States are affected, all of which may have as a common denominator, a chemical imbalance. The percent of this malady is  fifteen in men and eighty-five in women, although in some specific subgroups, such as the Gulf War Syndrome, as many as 80 percent of men have these problems. The Gulf War Syndrome has been much better defined in that almost 100 percent of the affected individuals had decrease of specific enzymes (N-acetyl-aspartate in one group and Ponaryl-esterace in another). These enzymes, when they are in sufficient amounts, protect the brain against sublethal doses of potential poisons that were there, but not officially deployed and also in our Governmental armamentarium, such as SARIN. A new variation of the older MRI and SPECT tests, the MRS (magnetic resonance spectroscopy) may more easily diagnose this one subset of the F word. I use syndrome and word interchangeably.

## A NEUROSOMATIC PROBLEM

Perhaps it is better to call this syndrome a *neuropsychoimmunoendocrinosomaticopathy*, or shorter, the Neurosomatic Syndrome, which carries all the potential tissue dysfunction.

Some scientists are "lumpers," lumping diseases together, others are "splitters," splitting disease into as many subcategories as possible. Any of the subdivisions of the neurosomatic syndrome, be it mitral valve prolapse, irritable bowel syndrome, allergies, fibromyalgia, migraine syndrome, multiple chemical sensitivity, dysautonomia, etc., can stand on their own and a case can be made that these could be a specific disease unto themselves. Depending on what specialists see the patient, they will have one or several of these diagnoses but they could also have symptoms in other organ systems as well as some fatigue. The underlying problems of what causes all these diseases will be discussed later. Much overlap exists and it is exceedingly rare that an individual has just one entity or subtype of the neurosomatic or F syndrome such as chronic fatigue syndrome alone, without some of the other diagnosis.

It was not too many years ago that doctors referred to these states as psychosomatic disease and let it go at that. Somatotization disorder, involving four different body sites usually begins before age 30 and lasts several years. This is defined by my psychiatrist colleagues as physical complaints without adequate cause. Additionally, hypochondriacal and malingering is a patient's display of what the psyche needs to be. Secondary gain, issues certainly need to be considered as well. These are not easily understood by most good primary care physicians. *Subsyndromal somatotization* is a diagnostic entity overused by many physicians, particularly psychiatrists who feel the problem is not real, but who are hesitant to really make a specific diagnosis. These, indeed, are somatic (bodily) complaints that do not fit into the niche of either specific psychiatric or medical diagnosis. There is still some validity to this medical entity that is very rare. Since the advent of the discovery of neurotransmitters and their interaction on our total body hormonal equilibrium, and the fact psychiatrists have to take much training in neurological diseases, subsyndromal somatotization is misused less and less. Therefore, I also use the term neurosomatic syndrome.

Researchers are developing new theories and novel therapies for the neurosomatic syndrome that, in the past, have been considered bizarre treatments such as detoxification of the intestines. The art rather than the science of medicine prevailed then, but now new facts are bringing out these as a more scientific approach. The treatment of these diseases might be amazingly simple or markedly convoluted. Hence, the patient and the doctor journey together down the path to amelioration and maybe even to a cure to their problem, which may take as short a time as ten minutes, after putting a few drops of medicine in the eye or as long as four years to get to the bottom of the problem. More about treatment later in this chapter.

Many patients refer to the neurosomatic diseases or the F word as a part of CFIDS (chronic fatigue immunodeficiency syndrome) or in children, to NIDS (neuroimmuno dysfunction syndrome), which may even border on autism. Some non-informed physicians refer to this problem as Dysthymia, Generalized Anxiety Disorder (GAD), Neuroticism or just a manipulative patient. As mentioned earlier, the Neurosomatic Syndrome has many subsets: Chronic Fatigue Syndrome; Fibromyalgia Syndrome; Myofascial Syndrome;

Irritable Bowel Syndrome (IBS); Mitral Valve Prolapse (MVP); Dysautonomia; Multiple Chemical Sensitivity Syndrome (MCSS); Exposure Syndrome (Sick Building Syndrome); Post Deployment Syndrome (Gulf War Syndrome); Nonspecific Skin Conditions; Migraine Headaches; Temporal Mandibular Disease (TMD); Premenstrual Syndrome (PMS); Allergy; Hypoglycemia; Genital Urinary Dysfunction; Food Intolerance; Chiari Syndrome; Weakness; Tremors; Dyspepsia; Vertigo; and some yet to be described syndromes. In an individual patient, there may be one or several of these sub syndromes at one time, or occurring in tandem.

## A CHEMICAL IMBALANCE

As in most diseases, there is an underlying genetic predisposition, such as an over-active immune system and Type A personality with superimposed environmental pressures that activate the F word. These include food allergies, nutritional deficiencies, toxin exposure, infection, and external stressors. Simply stated, these cause imbalance of the neuroendocrine system (the nervous system of both brain and peripheral nerves plus the glands that secrete hormones). The robust immune system, the system that fights not only infection, but, at times, even our own body such as seen in Lupus. Because of over damping of this same immune system, we are even more likely not able to fight an offending agent. A given stimulus, such as a viral infection, toxin, or an external stimulus activates the immune system to produce chemicals called cytokins and interleukins. Receptors for these chemicals have been found in the brain (hypothalamus), as well as most other tissues in our body. Specifically, there are pathways from the hypothalamus which go directly to the lymph nodes, and the endocrine system (thyroid, adrenal, pancreas, thymus, parathyroid). A feedback system from these glands by a neurotransmitter (a type of hormone such as serotonin or norepinephrine) back to the central nervous system (brain and spinal cord). For example, if there is an increased cytokin (an inflammatory chemical) with a viral infection, one would feel the usual muscle ache and tiredness that would normally resolve within several days. But, if abnormal messages get into the hypothalamus from an abnormally functioning brain because of external influences, the patient doesn't have the dampening out of the cytokins. The continual release of cytokins make one's symptoms go on and on and, hence, the muscle aches and fatigue continues.

In the automatic, or what we technically call the autonomic nervous system, there are two divisions, sympathetic and parasympathetic, which are usually in balance with the hypothalamus. It is not uncommon for the neurosomatic syndrome or the F Syndrome to have an inequality with one system overpowering the other. This is how I define dysautonomia. (See Figure 6-I, page 259.)

As its neurotransmitter, the sympathetic system has norepinephrine or noradrenaline, or in lay terms, just adrenaline. This prepares the body for flight or fight, or at times fright, causing the pupils to dilate for better vision, decreasing the blood supply to the intestines, increasing the heart rate to better supply the muscles to prepare us for the very active upcoming event. If things really get out of hand and we have severe body damage, then endorphins (another hormone) from our brain decrease our perception of pain. In contrast to this accelerator system, there is a breaking system with other neurotransmitters, such as acetylcholine. This allows us to return the blood supply to our intestines and other internal organs, slow our heart rate down, constrict our pupils and allow us to relax. However, if the breaking system is deficient, the poor person has a continued flight, fight, or fright feeling, despite the fact that the individual is neither fleeing nor fighting in a dangerous physical situation. Pseudo panic attacks such as these, are frequently misdiagnosed as coming from a psychiatric cause. But in these cases there is a true chemical neurotransmitter imbalance. This imbalance of these various processes (neurotransmitters, a mismatch of hormones, and non-dampening of the cytokin systems) allows for the symptoms and signs of these various subsets of the syndrome to be recognized. Symptoms are the patient's complaints and signs are the findings of the patient on examination.

There are a number of relatively simple maneuvers that will indicate which autonomic system is disturbed. A noninvasive technique performed with an electrocardiograph with a special software package can detail the part of the autonomic nervous system that is out of balance. This then can detail in the autonomic nervous system which of an how much two divisions sympathetic and parasympathetic are out of balance. Thus the Heart Rate Variability detailed on this type of EKG indicates which component needs to be augmented or decreased to balance the patient and to relieve the symptoms. This methodology that I use in my practice to fine tune the autonomic nervous system is indispensable in diagnosing and treating the F syndrome. Many simple blood tests can be helpful, such as the ALCAT (see page 57) to indicate food intolerance. There are more specific researched blood studies, such as a recently described test, 2, 5A (2, 5 synthetase/ribo nuclease L-pathway) which may be even diagnostic. According to Dr. Anthony L. Konaroff, editor in chief of *Harvard Health Publications*, this is a bio-marker that will put the disease on the scientific charts of orthodox medicine in that we will be able to do double-blind studies for both diagnosis and treatment. The 2, 5A molecule is made by the person's lymphocytes in response to a viral infection and helps to mount an antibody, antiviral defense. But the F patient makes an impotent, abnormal form of the 2, 5A. Therefore, the disease lingers until the immune system is improved by such maneuvers as toxin removal, better nutrition, hormonal balance, or a more restorative sleep. Also noted by Dr. Komaroff was a 26-fold higher circulating immune complex and an 8-fold higher level of IgG (two other blood tests). The 2, 5A is a test positive in 90 percent of patients with chronic fatigue syndrome and less than 10 percent of folks with just fibromyalgia.

# Fig. 6-I  Autonomic Nervous System in Balance

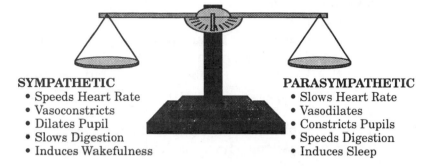

**SYMPATHETIC**
- Speeds Heart Rate
- Vasoconstricts
- Dilates Pupil
- Slows Digestion
- Induces Wakefulness

**PARASYMPATHETIC**
- Slows Heart Rate
- Vasodilates
- Constricts Pupils
- Speeds Digestion
- Induces Sleep

**NOPE** (Nitric Oxide Pain Element)

One cannot talk about these syndromes without some comment on Substance P in elemental pain and a malfunction of Nitric Oxide (NO). These are neurotransmitters, a chemical that makes nerves "talk" to one another, found in the brain and almost every peripheral tissue in our body. It is more than a coincidence that in the spinal fluid Substance P is two to three times higher in patients with these neurosomatic problems. Substance P is also increased most notably in the ligaments of fibromyalgia and contribute to the so-called tender points. According to Rheumatologists, 7 out of 11 need to be positive, or tender, to 8 pounds of pressure, compared to a central area such as at the base of the thumbnail to meet the criteria for the diagnoses of fibromyalgia. However, most physicians who really know fibromyalgia do not use this as a set of rules to "*rule in*" or "*rule out*" this disease. This should be for guidelines only. To make matters worse, a government agency, Center for Disease Control has both major and minor criteria for fibromyalgia. Five of these criteria are pain based, indicating there is too much Substance P in the organ or tissue. These are in addition to the tender points, muscle pain, joint pain, tender nodes, sore throat and headache. Substance P is *not* increased in psychiatric depression, but is increased in distress, both in humans and in non-human models. Patients with fibromyalgia just have too much Substance P and its accompaniment of pain. The remainder of this sub-chapter is extremely technical.

Brain molecules, such as NO, have been long identified along with their receptor. These include Opiates (endorphins), Gama Amino Buteric Acid (GABA), N-methyl D-aspartite (NMDA), Cortisol Releasing Factor (CRF), and Adrenal Cortical Trophic Hormone (ACTH). The last two are regulated by a feedback mechanism that does go awry with these medical problems. Scientists call these two an abnormal Hypothalamus-Pituitary Axis (HPA). An improperly tuned chemical feedback regulation stimulated by an external hormone or an abnormal stimulus in our brain causes the neurosomatic syndrome. Each neurohormone has a specific cellular receptor to which it connects and tells the cell what to or not to do. These receptors are sometimes overly active (up-regulated according to the medical jargon), or less active (down-regulated), depending on the activity of the receptors. Therefore, the same amount of hormone can produce more or less cellular activity. The most substantially researched neurotransmitter is norepinephrine, which is abnormally low and/or its receptor is down-regulated. This is manifested in the heart as in MVP or in the arteries, causing NMH (Neurally Mediated Hypotension) or in the muscle effecting a decreased exercise tolerance.

Nociception is a neurochemical process by which a pain signal is transmitted from the periphery to the Central Nervous System (brain and spinal cord). This process begins with a noxious stimulus that distorts or damages tissue, and leads to increased synthesis and release of endogenous inflammatory chemical products. NMDA receptors cause the release of substance P, which binds mainly with neurokinin-1 (NK-1) receptor molecules. Substance P also results in the release of calcitonin gene-related peptide (CGRP) and neurokinin, and the generation of a certain dependent prostaglandin that initiates transmission of the pain signal to the brain. The resulting activation of NMDA receptor sites and release of substance P leads to a hyperexcitability of CNS neurons, which is known as *central sensitization*. It lowers the threshold of excitability, which leads to the unmasking of normally silent nerve cells and the sensitization of other spinal neurons. Also, substance P can extend in the dorsal horn to sensitize neurons at some distance from the initial stimulus. This leads to expansion of pain beyond the area expected or in medical jargon, *enlargement of peripheral receptive fields*. There are two types of spinal neurons involved in central sensitization, a nociceptive-specific neuron and wide-dynamic-range (WDR) neuron. These respond to both nociceptive and nonnociceptive afferent stimuli. After sensitization, WDR neurons will respond to nonnoxious stimuli before sensitization. As a result, nonnoxious sensations, such as light touch, are experienced as pain. Thus, nonpainful impulses are noted as painful (allodynia), and nociceptive nerve impulses are perceived as even more painful (hyperalgesia). The wind-up phenomenon may explain how persistent stimulation of peripheral nerves can lead to a disproportionate upregulation of nervous activity, resulting in hyperalgesia, allodynia, and persist pain.

An increase in nitric oxide (NO) during immune activation lowers overall adrenal output and will cause the same clinical picture now evident in chronic fatigue syndrome, myofascial syndrome, and fibromyalgia. NO not only lowers cortisol, but other hormones like aldosterone, DHEA, pregnenolone and adrenal like secretions. This leads to a lower adrenal output (defect in pituitary-hypothalamus feedback relationship). The evidence in CFS and at times its little sisters, FMS and MFS, all point to a reduced ACTH response to specific stimuli. Since NO is a neurotransmitter, it does have a receptor on which to act. It is these receptors that are upregulated by an insult to our body such as infections, chemical stress, or physical stress. Upregulated nitric oxide due to hyperimmunity and with another toxic gas, carbon monoxide alters hypothalmus-pituitary function and creates the exact same pattern now evidenced in the chronic fatigue syndrome.

Over production (up regulation) of NO in the brain causes the specific neuro hormone N-methyl-D-aspartate (NMDA) to have too much activity. Gama Amino Buteric Acid (GABA) offsets NDMA and it is the relationship of the NDMA to GABA that makes the brain (and the body) function correctly or abnormally. Many compounds offset the GABA/NMDA relationship both directly and indirectly. These include simple molecules (magnesium) to more complex (aspirin) to hormones (cortisone) to active drugs (Klonopin, Ritalin, etc.). This will be discussed later under treatment.

## INFECTION

Another distinct cause of many people with the F Syndrome is that the immune system is not regulated and is either over stimulated or depressed. Opportunistic infections such as yeast, fungi, parasites and smaller, more fastidious germs such as certain strains of chlamydia, mycoplasma, primordial life forms, and viruses could cause the problem. As discussed, our immune cells have too much of the enzyme, Rnase-L, which makes our cells sick. They actually pull the trigger on a gun loaded by immuno suppressors in a genetically susceptible individual. Research, published in October 1999, found mycoplasma DNA in 70 percent of patients with the F word, compared to 9 percent of a normal population. Mycoplasmas are a primitive, slow-growing type of bacteria, hard to culture, and susceptible to only a few antibiotics. In certain chemical states characterized by chronic oxidative stress such as the F Syndrome, there is a mild acidosis, which favors the growth of certain germs. Almost 100 years ago, Gunther Enderlein discovered primordial life forms not only in human tissue but also in the blood. These are readily observed with a high resolution phase-contrast and dark field microscope in a fresh, whole blood slide. These organisms feed the oxidative flame, regenerating even more oxidative free radicals and causing the continued kindling of the F Syndrome's vicious downward spiral. More research needs to be done to prove a cause and effect with these and other organisms. However, doctors can now formulate a treatment plan for some of the poor folks who have this disease.

# A PAIN IN THE NECK

In a small percentage of folks with the neurosomatic syndrome (3-8 percent), the problem is anatomic. The Chiari Syndrome is a congenital abnormality with the natural opening at the base of the skull being smaller than normal. This could also be acquired later in life by arthritis narrowing this canal (cervical stenosis). The nervous tissue is being pushed down this opening by pressure above such a persistent coughing with resultant pressure on the autonomic nerves. The impaction of the hard bones on the soft nerves hence causes dysfunction. This is associated with hyperalgesia allodynia and dysautonomia.

To confirm this diagnosis, a neurologic abnormality such as defined by anatomical weakness, loss of muscle mass, abnormal nerve conduction, or loss of reflexes should be documented first, then an MRI performed. If this then shows the Chiari defect, a knowledgeable neurosurgeon with lots of experience should review the case. These include as Dan Huffey, M.D. at the Chicago Institute of Neurosurgery or Michael Rosner at the University of Alabama in Birmingham. A neurosurgical procedure then would cure the patient.

Chiropractic may help here, not only by pain relieving of back and extremities, but also by giving more energy to a fatigue patient. In particular, the Grostic technique can greater help some of these folks without, but particularly those with the Chiari malformation. John Grostic was a chiropractor who discovered this technique and his son, John Grostic, Jr. who is an engineer and a chiropractor who refined the procedure. Special x-ray views are done in the chiropractic office and the "malalignment" is calculated. The patient is asked to lay down on a 5-inch high table with the neck having no support. By putting minimal pressure in the specific angle on the neck, the pressure is taken off the underlying nervous tissue and the F Syndrome could go into remission. Not all chiropractors, even though they profess to, know the procedure or can do it well. There is a national registry of Grosetic practitioners. I have seen success.

# MYOFASCIAL SYNDROME (MFS)

Myofascial Syndrome is localized musculoskeletal pain usually associated with generalized aching, stiffness or fatigue. Unlike fibromyalgia, it occurs slightly more in men than women. Occasionally an underlying initial insult causes the problem. This may be overstressing the muscle and/or tendon, trauma of the musculoskeletal group, giving a slight interruption of the nervous vascular transmission to that unit. Subsequent to one of these insults, there is recurrence of pain in that muscle and tendon. At times, the pain arises insidiously with no known precipitating event. Referred pain is common and there is a trigger point some distance from where the actual tenderness is. Do not confuse *tender* points seen in cases of fibromyalgia with a *trigger* point, as many doctors do. For example, touching over the scapula will cause pain in the arm. The scapular area is the trigger point. The so-called neural arc theory has been invoked to explain why these people have continuous pain. A reflex system goes from the muscle through nerves to the spinal cord and then back again to the muscle. A release into the muscle of Substance P causes the pain. The sensation is transmitted through an incoming pathway (the sympathetic nerve) to the spinal cord. Then from the spinal cord to the muscle again, causing the release of more substance P occurs, which again stimulates the neural pathway and a vicious cycle is set up. The pain is usually deep and aching and may become multi-regional. There may also be a painful restriction of the range of motions.

Specifically with treatment or nonspecifically with time, this reflex arc becomes dampened and the symptoms resolve. However, minimal stimulus such as a repeated small bout of trauma will "turn on" this reflex arc again with the release of more substance P, causing a recurrence of the symptomatology. Some people have this problem, and once it starts, intermittently, have it throughout their lives. Many patients with low back pain and some with chronic neck pain have a myofascial syndrome. It can be one (unilateral) or both (bilateral) sides of the body.

Localized physical therapy such as the alteration of heat and cold, a special spectrum light, magnets, ultrasound, electrical stimulation, TENS (Transdermal Electrical Neuro Stimulation), and restorative sleep may be of help. I sometimes apply a technique learned from Janet Travell, MD (President Kennedy's physician, who advised a rocking chair for his bad back) called "The Spray and Stretch Technique". A vapor coolant spray, ethyl chloride, is employed. This is sprayed from the origin of the tendon to the belly of the muscle and then to the opposite tendon back and forth every half inch. At the same time, I stretch the muscle tendon unit. I have achieved immediate success. In some cases I use Neural Therapy (injection of a local anesthetic lidocaine) or a shot of cortisone, injected into the pseudo-inflamed area. In other cases, I do proliferative therapy, a solution of Sarapin (a homeopathic remedy from the pitcher plant listed in the Physicians Desk Reference) and a concentrated glucose solution (12.5 percent). The fluid is injected deeply into the ligaments. This causes proliferation of the collagen (glue tissue) within the tendon of the involved muscle group and this tightens the "bands" for the proper function of the muscle-tendon joint unit. The procedure can be likened to tightening up a lose rubber band on a child's toy by tying a knot in it.

A cousin of the myofascial syndrome, some physicians feel, is osteoarthritis, caused by the loosened ligament around a joint. The joint is no longer stabilized, and there is excess "play" in that joint. Since the bones are not seated well, it wobbles with their every movement, causing excess stress on various parts of the joint surface. The joint cartilage responds by growing bigger at the point of stress, and hence, it becomes asymmetric. Still later, the bone underlying the cartilage becomes thickened and thus deformed. According to this theory, this osteoarthritis is not a joint or a bone disease, but a ligament problem. If one treats the ligaments early, there may be no osteoarthritis.

# FIBROMYALGIA SYNDROME (FMS)

Although there is much overlap with eighty-five percent of patients with CFS having FMS and thirty percent of FMS patients having CFS and both having MFS. FMS is a disease unto itself. Fibromyalgia Syndrome is the most common cause of chronic diffuse pain that I see in my practice. Although well described by Sir William Osler in 1892, this problem has been around as long as mankind has walked our planet. In the past, it has been called lumbago, rheumatism, fibromyositis, fibritis and hemodynia (pain where the blood flows, i.e. all over the body). Allodynia occurs in FMS. This is an alteration of pain perception in which a normally painless stimulus is rendered painful. An example is ones clothes touching them, which is disturbing. More common is hyperalgesia, where slight stimuli in the nociceptive pain receptors are perceived as much more painful, hence the tender points. These result from the biochemical abnormalities, as noted earlier, associated with serotonin, substance P, neuroadrenaline, NO, GABA, NMDA, Adenosine Tri-Phosphate (ATP), altered glucose metabolism, Insulin-like Growth Factor (IGF-1), hyaluronidase, as well as a disordered regulation of various adrenal and thyroid hormonal production and their receptors.

Clinical features of FMS are that of diffuse aching, non-specific muscle stiffness, numbness, fatigue, sleep disturbances, and tension type headaches. Inclement weather, such as a new front coming in, will cause, in some cases, a flare-up of symptoms. It usually starts at age twenty with peak incidence at age forty (average age is twenty-five). It is estimated that between five and twelve percent of the population may have this problem. There is a family predisposition to fibromyalgia. It is seen in twenty times as many women as men. Some doctors, today, use the term "psychogenic rheumatism", indicating that it's in the patient's mind. With this I could not disagree more, as noted earlier. Patients who are told this, should either educate their doctor or find another one. Contrary to CFS, FMS without CFS patients note little, if any neuro-psychiatric symptoms other than if having a painful life that can cause real depression.

Although not well documented, I suspect that Fibromyalgia Syndrome is really the manifestation of 15 to 20 underlying problems. In the year 2100, we will know the specific pieces of the puzzle, but in 2001, we will discuss it as one disease. It is only with time and response to certain nebulous therapies that we are working out some of the nuances and, hence, subtypes of this clinical mystery will unfold. We have dissected out many other diseases already from FMS, such as the mutation of the cytochrome b gene of mitochondrial DNA as described by Dr. Andrew Lloyd in a 1999 *New England Journal* article and more will be forth coming.

As mentioned earlier, tender, not trigger points are said to be the most specific diagnostic criteria of this disease. The American College of Rheumatology has mapped out 18 tender points, of which the doctor needs to find at least 11 to be "diagnostic." The examiner usually touches them with his finger, but will, occasionally, use a specific instrument, called a dolorimeter, to elicit a response. Why these points are tender is controversial, but we do know that there is an increase of a chemical substance P, as discussed earlier. Biopsies of these tender points reveal no clear-cut abnormality under a regular or even an electron microscope. There is some data to suggest that a local decrease in blood flow with a diminished amount of high energy phosphate (ATP) exists in these regions. Increased cerebral blood flow to certain areas of the brain to include the thalamus and caudate nucleus have been measured by a single photon emission and computed tomography indicating, a generalized alteration of the pain threshold (allodynia). PET and neurospect scans have shown similar abnormalities. There is a clear-cut abnormality in the neuroendocrine system with increased pain, an abnormality in sleep and mood. Altered levels of serotonin and norepinephrine have been documented deep in the brain. Growth hormone, coming from the pituitary gland, is also decreased in many of these patients. However, the bottom line is that these folks have a decreased threshold to pain in potentially all their tissues, be it heart, intestines, skin, muscles, blood vessels, causing various manifestations of their disease.

Sleep disturbance has been long suspected in many patients with fibromyalgia Some of these are primary sleep abnormalities such as periodic involuntary limb motion and sleep apnea. Others are nonspecific and the patient is said to have a *nonrestorative sleep*. Frequent awakenings may be noticed by the patient. We also know that medications that enhance the quality of sleep help. The deepest stage of sleep where it is the most difficult for a patient to be aroused, is markedly decreased. During this type of sleep, in which there is rapid eye movement (REM), most of the muscle restorative function is said to exist. Growth hormone has been noted to be released during REM sleep and hence is reduced, proportional to the amount of REM sleep obtained. Treatment of this FMS will be discussed in greater detail at the end of this chapter, but it is assuring that it is not life threatening and there is no deformity expected. Although one may not ever be cured, there is definitely help. Sometimes, telling a patient this alone makes him feel better.

## CHRONIC FATIGUE SYNDROME (CFS)

As mentioned earlier in this chapter, CFS has been around ever since humans have come into being, and it may be present in animals as well. Postdeployment syndromes such as *De Costa Syndrome*, described during the Civil War, *Shell Shock* in WW I, *Neurocirculatory Asthenia* in WW II, *Post Traumatic Stress Syndrome* of the Vietnam War and the *Gulf War Syndrome*, recently, are part of what we call Chronic Fatigue Syndrome today. In that it may have an immunologic factor as stated, sometimes referred to as CFIDS (Chronic Fatigue Immune Deficiency Syndrome), or in children, NIDS (Neruoimmuno Dysfunction Syndrome). Actually, there have been outbreaks of this malady, documented by the U.S. Public Health Service, in the 1930s and 1950s. It gained prominence by the public in mid 1980s when Dr. Paul Cheny described the epidemic at Lake Taho. It became a rec-

## Table 6-I
## Evolution of Diagnosis in Chronic Fatigue Syndrome

| MAJOR CRITERIA | 1988 (CDC*) | 1994 (CDC*) | 2001 (J.E.B.**) | 2010 (ALL***) |
|---|---|---|---|---|
| Specific blood studies | + | - | - | + |
| Down regulation of B12 receptor | + | - | - | + |
| Rnase-L positivity | - | - | + | + |
| New onset | + | + | + | + |
| Decrease growth hormone | + | - | - | + |
| No previous history | + | + | - | - |
| Does not resolve with bed rest | + | + | + | + |
| Activity reduction >50% | | | + | + |
|   lasting > 6 months | + | + | - | + |
| Exclude all illnesses | + | + | - | - |
| Exclude all psychiatric disorders | + | ± | + | - |
| Exclude eating disorders | + | + | + | + |

| MINOR CRITERIA | 1988 (CDC*) | 1994 (CDC*) | 2001 (J.E.B.**) | 2010 (ALL***) |
|---|---|---|---|---|
| Autonomic dysfunction | - | - | + | + |
| Low systolic pressure | - | - | + | + |
| Documented fingerprint destruction | - | - | + | + |
| Subnormal temperature | - | - | + | + |
| Sore throat | + | + | + | + |
| Painful lymph nodes | + | + | + | + |
| Generalized weakness | + | - | + | + |
| Muscle discomfort (pain) | + | + | + | + |
| Prolonged fatigue after exercise | + | + | + | + |
| 20 point drop in BP from sitting to standing | - | - | + | + |
| Generalized (new) headaches | + | + | + | + |
| Migratory arthralgias | + | + | - | + |
| Neuropsychiatric complaints (impaired memory or concentration) | + | + | + | + |
| Sleep disorders (unrefreshing sleep) | + | + | + | + |
| Acute onset | + | - | - | + |
| Documented low-grade fever | + | - | + | + |
| Documented nonexudative pharyngitis | + | - | - | + |
| Documented palpable or tender lymph nodes | + | - | - | + |
| Failed equilibrium test | - | - | + | + |
| Inability to hold breath | - | - | + | + |

* Communicable Disease Center    **J.E. Block, M.D.    ***All

ognized disorder in 1988 when a case definition was developed under the auspices of the U.S. Center for Disease Control and Prevention. Specific criteria with major and minor points were concluded by a consensus of scientists. Although these criteria are used in research work, most astute physicians do not use these, and even researchers change them from time to time. (See Table 6-I.) Perhaps in the year 2010 all will agree with the criteria. They will be much more specific with the symptoms superimposed on the signs and documented with a laboratory test. Not only that, the specific disease subset will be easily treated.

In a study published in the *American Journal of Medicine* in September of 1998, Dr. Andrew Lloyd stated that in any given population, fourteen percent of the people feel "tired out" and 2.2 percent feel weak. As noted in Table I, one needs to have these symptoms for six months or more. Many times, the patients can tell you the exact date their problems started. For example, one of my patients stated he was well until three years ago in February when he had a respiratory infection that lasted a little longer than usual. During that time, he felt extremely fatigued. He got a little better, only to have a relapse, with the fatigue and difficulty in thinking, which has been continuous ever since that time!

Many people are unable to get out of bed, let alone go to work or function as a mother or a wife. Patients vacillate between good days and weeks and bad. However, most days of even the good weeks are not without the patient feeling drained. Individuals who have led a robust life in the recent past are now confined to their home and sometimes to bed.

The triad of CFS symptoms are energy, brain, and pain. When the brain is involved, this is primarily a cognitive and not a significant mood problem. Of the neuropsychic phenomena which happens in ninety-nine percent of the cases there are problems in processing short term memory (particularly auditory), sensory information overload (light too bright, noise too loud), word searching, multi-tasking problems and spatial disorganization. Of course, there are secondary mood disturbances in 60 percent of the cases which include mild depression, anxiety and lability of mood. The pain is that of FMS or MFS.

The Physical Examination shows immune activation characterized by enlarged, painful lymph nodes, particularly in the neck in ninety percent of patients. As many as eighty percent of the patients have an arc of purple over the soft palate. This phenomena is also seen in twenty percent of normals and is related to activation of the small lymphoid tissue within the soft palate. Additionally, there is an elevated temperature in twenty-five percent with the morning temperatures greater than 99.4 degrees and in another thirty-five percent a subnormal temperature. Brain injury is noted in that if one tests the equilibrium, almost ninety-four percent would fail. These include closing the eyes and standing up even in the most mild cases. The so-called tandem stance test with one leg straight out while the other foot is flat against the ground is abnormal (this is the same test police may do when suspected of drunken driving). Additionally, the deep tendon reflexes are changed with an over-active reflex in the knees and heels and decreased ones in the upper extremities. Metabolic disturbances are noted in that the ninety-five percent of the patients cannot hold their breath more than 15 seconds. Anatomically, fifty percent of the patients have fingerprint destruction of each hand under the nail and slowly working its way to the first central swirl. This starts first at the little finger and then next to the ring finger and gradually involves all the fingers. In 50-100 percent of patients, there is a low systolic blood pressure (less than 110) and when one goes from a sitting to standing position there is a 20 point drop and greater than a 20 pulse rise. Very rarely do we see hypertension. Many former hypertensive patients become normalized.

The evolution of CFS includes three phases to include Phase One, the *trigger* (usually viral infection); Phase Two, the *triad* (fatigue, brain dysfunction, pain); and Phase Three, the *dynamic injury*. The trigger phase usually presents as a usual viral infection with flu-like achiness, swollen glands, generalized aches and pains that goes on and on. In thirty percent of the cases, there has been another presentation such as a head injury, an overwhelming stressful situation with perhaps exposure to a toxin (Gulf War Syndrome), or an extreme physical insult such as an automobile accident, being hit by lightening, or major surgery with complications. In general, the trigger phase lasts six months, but has been as short as two weeks to as long as six years.

In the triad phase is that the patient becomes more fatigued, the brain becomes involved with neuropsychiatric phenomena and muscle pains increase. This lasts eight to twelve years and goes on to the third phase. Sometimes, there is a stuttering evolution from the second to the third phase. Patients in the third phase say they are doing so much better, they can think better and their pain is less, but they know their limitations. They feel that if they push the envelope too far, they crash. If they stay within their boundaries, they do okay. However, the boundaries keep changing and the patient occasionally does over step the line and has to pay for this with more symptomatology.

The underlying problem that occurs in Phase One is an immunocellular abnormality characterized by the viral induced chemical called Rnase-L. People with a very strong immune system are more likely to get CFS. Phase Two is a cellular toxicity with injury perhaps due to xenobiotics. Phase Three is injury to the central nervous system and is associated with DNA gene rearrangement. Following Phase Three, there may be a recovery phase and indeed, 50 percent do get better from Phase Three according to a recent study, but it may be years or decades and the improvement is gradual. In that this is a relatively recent disease for long follow up, research has not been done on what happens to the other 50 percent I assume that half of these will get better in even more decades to come and the remainder may get worse. Teenagers seem to recover sooner and those that are mentally very positive have a faster recovery. On the other hand, the Personality Type A is really clobbered with their disease and are frequently in a situation where they just cannot cope that their "spirit is willing, but their flesh is weak."

Although I will discuss more about treatment at the end of this chapter, let me mention some things peculiar to CFS. In 1996, Mark Demitrack M.D., described neuromediated hypotension (NMH). This was treated with additional salt and, in some extreme cases, Florinef, a drug that increases sodium retention. Dr. Robin McKenzie published an article in the *Journal of American Medicine Association* (Sept. 30, 1998) and suggested CFS may be due to adrenal fatigue. Bearing this in mind, low dose hydrocortisone has shown to be effective for some of these patients. Autonomic tests have been done by me on some patients which included a tilt table and hand grip rest. I have abandoned these procedures because they were found to be of no help, and use the EKG heart rate variability test. I have used the treatment of steroids empirically. I give five mg of Prednisone in the morning and half that at noon. At these small doses, this inexpensive drug is safe for the average person, even taking it for years. It is true that Prednisone is a form of cortisone, but has obtained a bad name because of the abuse of it by physicians in the past. Since adrenaline may play a large role in CFS, an adrenaline like drugs, such as amphetamine, or Ritalin has been used with some success. However, these are addictive, and I try not to use it in that the side effects of treatment may be worse than the disease. On the other hand, the newly released drug, Robetexin, a SNRI (Selective Norepinephine Reaceptake Inhibitor) has helped some patients. Of interest, in fifty percent of the cases taking three to four-5 grain aspirins at once at the time of extreme fatigue will rev up a CFS victim's energy for 30-40 minutes in most cases. Exercise, starting very gradually and increased weekly, very often helps CFS. Exercise up-regulates the norepinephrine receptors so that muscles will function better and better. It takes three or four months to work up to a strenuous exercise program involving both aerobic (running, biking, etc.), as well as anaerobic (weight lifting), but if the per-

# Table 6-II

# Preparations Useful in the F Syndrome

Please see Chapter Five for details on some of these and of other therapeutics.

## Nonprescription Supplements

Alpha-ketoglutarate

Amino acids*

Androdiestine

Aspartame (Nutrasweet)

Aspirin

Beta Glucan (1,3/1,6)

Betaine Hydrochloride/Pepsin

Bioflavinoids (especially quercetin)

Blue-green algae

Butyric acid

Capascin

Carnitine

Chondroitin sulfate

Coenzyme Q10

CMO

Colostrum

DLPA

DHEA

DMSO

EPA

Essential fatty acids**

Glucosamine

Glutamine

Glycine Powder

Gookinaid ERG

Herbs***

LEM****

Malic Acid

Melatonin

Minerals****

MSM (methyl sulfur methane)

NADH (Nada™)

Niacinamide

Probioplex

Probiotics

pycnogenol

Royal Jelly

SAMe

Vitamins (B12, B6 and E)

* 5HTP, GLA, Glutathione, glycine Lysine, taurine

** Flax, borage, Evening primrose oil

*** Astralgus, boswella, cat's claw, ginseng, ginkgo biloba, grapefruit, green tea, echinacea, licorice, St. John's Wort, Sambucol, Valerian

**** Lentimus edodes mycelum (an immature shitachi mushroom)

*****Calcium, lithium, magnesium, sodium, zinc

## Table 6-III
## Generic Prescription Drugs

| | |
|---|---|
| Acetozolamide | Naphazoline eye drops |
| Ampligen | Nimodopine |
| Amitriptyline | Nitroglycerin |
| Baclofen | Ondansetron |
| Calcitonin | Paroxetine |
| Doxepin | Pindolol |
| Gabapentin | Prednisone |
| Hyaluronidase | Propanolol |
| Hydralazine | Roboxatine* |
| Human Growth Hormone | Sertraline |
| Kutapressin | Sumatriptan |
| Lidocaine | Tiagabine |
| Lithium | Tizanidine |
| Methadone | Tramadol |
| Methylarginine* | Venlafaxine |
| Modafinil | Zaleplon |
| | Zalpidem |

Compounding pharmacies are very useful, not only in the knowledge of the F Syndrome but they will make you any prescribed preparation authorized by your physician. Your nearest one can be obtained by calling 1-800-333-4622.

*FDA approval pending

son, particularly with CFS, over steps their bounds, they will pay for it in increased symptoms for days to come. Fibromyalgia patients benefit more from exercise than chronic fatigue. Limbic exercises, which stimulate the center of the brain, such as Yoga and Tai Chi are particularly helpful. These improve hypothalamic as well as somatic functioning. Since there is a daily variation of symptoms, later I will give you my most recent regime.

To work up a patient, a battery of lab tests are sometimes ordered. In scientific literature, patients with CFS have low levels of killer cells. This does not correlate well with the disease, similarly checking for various viruses, such as Epstein Barr. We stopped doing these tests 12 years ago when the literature suggested it was *not* due to mononucleosis alone, but a myriad of viruses or other infections and it probably is too late to treat the virus anyhow. Over the years, I have done tests for latent herpes virus and even treated some patients with the herpes suppressor drug, Acyclovir, without success and, therefore, I no longer test or treat for this or other viruses. Recently human growth hormone deficiency has been implicated in both fibromyalgia on CFS and blood studies for this to include IGF-1 could be done.

Functional studies to include the MRI, SPECT and PET may be positive and ordered in some medical practices. These are expensive and for the most part useless unless one wants to make sure there is no underlying disease missed, such as the Chiari Syndrome (see page 263) or multiple sclerosis. On the other hand, a special EEG study may be helpful if I plan to use neurobiofeedback (see page 279). I used to do but have abandoned an exhaustive treadmill exercise, looking at its effect on cognitive function and post exercise malaise. As mentioned above, the EKG heart rate variability test gives not only the diagnosis of dysautonomia, but an idea as to if the current treatment plan is efficacious.

## Specific Treatment Philosophy

Like all other diagnoses and treatments, education as to the true nature of the disease, what we as physicians can do and, more importantly, *what we cannot do*, is explained to the patient. Patients play the biggest role in their therapy. Since all patients are different, and the disease process is not the same in all individuals, what works in one does not work in another. I encourage my patients to read, go to seminars and use the Web. It is true art, based on science, depending on the patient's presentation and profile as well as the doctor's knowledge and the acceptance of Integrative Medicine and how well he or she keeps up with the literature. There is no magic bullet, and it may take months or years for the patient to get better. Usually, several therapies are given at once, and a treatment protocol is developed *specifically* for a *specific* patient. The longer the duration, the longer the frustration of the patient, the more maladaptive habits are formed, and the more difficult the disease is to treat. Secondary gains from their illness have surfaced and disability issues need to be considered. After five years of inability to work and insurance or Social Security payments almost ready to start, does that patient *really* want to get better? Certainly she did five years ago, but what about now? Without the patient's 100 percent cooperation, treatment is doomed to fail.

At this point in time, the F Syndrome (CFS/FMS/MFS) is a group of diseases all having much in common. In years to come, science may tease out specific diseases and then we can treat them specifically. In the last decade, major depression has been easily separated from the F Syndrome by giving an antidepressive. After six weeks, this subgroup of patients were markedly improved. Certainly, with the frustrations of having a poorly defined disease in a patient who looks healthy but feels miserable, the person can end up with depression. This is a secondary depression. There may be some improvement in these patients with antidepressives, but not to the point as if these symptoms were all due to a primary depression.

The treatment is geared to the phase of the disease of which the patient has. This is particularly true with CFS, but since there is much overlap between MFS, CFS and FMS, it may help all of these. As noted earlier, most CFS patients have fibromyalgia, but a smaller percent of FMS people have CFS. With CFS, demarcation between phases is not very sharp or clear cut. Folks transition from phase to phase; at times is seamlessly and at other times there is a definite change, and still others it is one day in phase II and the next day in phase III. Phase I treatment is directed towards too much of the cellular enzyme, Rnase-L, which functions as our cellular mechanism to destroy foreign invaders such as a virus. But, in CFS patients the immune system is so revved up that the cell malfunctions. If this goes on too long, it affects our intestines and liver. These organs do not detoxify properly and the patient transcends into stage II, which is characterized by xenotoxicity. For phase I, antimicrobial or antiviral therapy may be used, but this is just a shot in the dark. Frequently, by the time the disease is recognized, it is too late. However, we can decrease the incidence of CFS by giving proper respect to all infection. In particular, proper rest and nutrition during the very early stage. Drugs, such as Ampligen, have a role in this phase. Immune modulation by supplements, such as antioxidants (vitamins C and E), sometimes help. In stage II, in which the cell has too much acid (intracellular acidosis), we try to normalize the acid. Drugs, such as Diamox (Acetozolamide), or special breathing to hold in temporarily more carbon dioxide helps in many patients. Diamox, as well as the breathing, enhances a natural cellular enzyme (2-3 DPG) to neutralize the intracellular acid. As described on a tape by Andrew Wiel, first breathe in for four seconds through the nose, hold for seven seconds, and then breathe out against a resistance for eight seconds. The resistance could be pursed lips, a twirled tongue, or through a slightly pinched nosed with the mouth closed. This procedure is repeated ten times in a row, five times a day (five sets of ten reps). Initially, some patients feel as if they are going to pass out and the procedure can be modified i.e. less time of holding breath, less reps, less sets and then gradually increase as they feel better and better.

Most folks with CFS have a marked decrease of their fluid volume. Many patients drink lots of water, which is needed, but because of their over abundance of citrate being leached out of their sick cells, it washes out the all important mineral, magnesium. The lack of magnesium makes the blood vessels constrict and adds insult to injury. Pentahydrate (page 100) or Gookinaid ERG will combat this fluid and mineral loss. (Mr. Gookin was a marathon winner in the early '80s and first developed this drink for runners). Gookinaid is absorbed rapidly through the stomach and is not urinated out rapidly like other fluids (water, pop, juices, etc). Magnesium supplements can also be given orally. There are many products on the market, both in drug and health food stores, and four to five time the usual dose is recommended with Slomag (64 mg) take four or five a day. Do the same with Mag Oxide (400 mg) if you choose that product. No prescription is needed for magnesium. I also recommend intramuscular injections of magnesium, taurine, and large doses of $B_{12}$. In phase II, I recommend autonomic nervous system regulation that can be done with gradual exercises to include Yoga and Tai Chi. Rebound exercise, bodywork, and neurobiofeedback help the latter in particular for the neuropsychic phenomena as brainfog, mood lability, memory, multitasks, and spatial organizations. I have advised the EEG neurobiofeedback for returning sensibility in these poor folks' brain.

## Neurobiofeedback

The human mind is capable of altering the autonomic nervous system by a mechanism that is not entirely conscious. With an EEG and modern computerized technology, one can observe their own brain waves on a monitor instantaneously, called 'real time.' Also, it is possible for a person to concentrate on certain patterns and amplitude of the brain waves and *modify* them by intent. By remodeling the brain waves in specified ways, it is possible for people to *improve* their brain function and treat certain disease states. This technique can help people with spasticity (strokes, multiple sclerosis, and cerebral palsy), addictions, tremors (movement diseases), post-polio syndrome, ADHD, migraine, head injury, depression, seizure disorders, anxiety and the F Syndrome. In a recent study, approximately 90% of children taking Ritalin, for ADD/ADHD, have been able to dispense with that, educational scores have increased, behavior has improved by every measure, and parental satisfaction has also improved.

The technique is fairly simple. Electrodes are placed strategically on the head to monitor the underlying electrical activity of brain function. These may or may not be the locations used for a conventional EEG. The computer is programmed to filter out the unwanted frequencies and voltages and leaves the desired **alpha**, **beta**, **theta**, or **delta** waves. In addition to the graphic display on the monitor, the wave noises are concurrently transmitted via earphones so the patient receives both visual and auditory stimuli.

An EEG is a composite of the above mentioned four waves. In CFS, there is a predominance of the pre-sleep **theta** rather than the **beta** waves. The latter is typical of an alert individual by knowing the feeling of a given wave and by concentrating on what produces the **beta** waves an individual can, after being trained, commute the **theta** waves to **beta** at will. Clinically, the fatigue and brain fog will dissipate. If it returns later, the person again can change its state within two seconds. Several training sessions lasting one hour are needed and then the patient, with the aid of the equipment, can practice two to three times a week for two months, and have a "cure" for the problem. The equipment costs between fifteen to thirty thousand dollars and is made by several companies. Looking at the literature, I like the device endorsed by Margaret Ayers. She is a Ph.D. psychologist who, in 1975, started publishing her research while at UCLA. Initially, she worked with head trauma and stroke patients, but now these procedures are used mostly for ADD and ADHD, although they work well for the F word.

In Phase III, CFS folks have learned their boundaries and although they keep changing, the person has developed an idea of where they are. The patient has also been educated in much of the additional therapies discussed in this chapter that can be used for acute and chronic disability. They, with their health care worker, feel optimistic that they are going to eventually win the war with CFS although they may be still loosing an occasion battle.

Tizanidine HCI (Zanaflex ™) is another option. Its site of action is both in the spinal cord and in the brain at the adrenal active locus of the Caeruleus. Its FDA prescribed use is for muscle spacisity such as in multiple sclerosis or stroke. But because of its anti-nociceptive activity it decreases unneeded pain perception. There is no tolerance or addiction compared to the opiates or benzothiopines such as Xanax™. It is a safe drug. Five percent of patients will have elevated liver enzymes within the first six months and this blood test will need to be monitored. There is a chance of a drop in blood pressure, but the common side effect is a dose related sedation and dry mouth. The 4mg pill is scored so it can be broken into quarters and from 1mg three times a day slowly until a maximum of 32mg a day are given. I back down the dose if there are side effects of too much fatigue, dry mouth, or a significant drop in blood pressure and give it even lower and slower.

Adjunctive treatment for any of the phases is lifestyle adjustments by limiting commitments; tell family and community of the ailment in a deliberate non-solicitous way. One may have to change work style, profession, or consider a transient retirement. A healthy diet is recommended. Sometimes I advise staying away from night shade vegetables (tomatoes, potatoes, green peppers, etc.). Occasionally, I use the ALCAT or the Great Smokies food study for determination of food intolerance (see page 57). Digestive enzymes and detoxification procedures are recommended.

In the pathways to self-healing such as stress reduction, conscious beliefs and attitudes, medication and spiritual involvement is necessary. As mentioned earlier, the more religious activities the person performs, the better it is. There are ways to provide protection to the nervous system, particularly the neurotransmitters. For the NMDA blockers, magnesium and taurine, as well as the antihistamines such as Doxepin may be helpful. For the GABA enhancing receptors, Klonopin day and night, Neurontin at night, or day, and kava-kava in the day and valerian root at night.

Because the disease will affect our genes and DNA, I recommend antioxidant vitamins, bioflavonoids, coenzyme $Q_{10}$, lipoic acid, essential fatty acids and occasional Melatonin at night. In that homocystine is elevated in the central nervous system, folic acid, Pyridoxine ($B_6$), Cyanocobolamine ($B_{12}$), taurine, trimethyl glycine (TMG) and SAM-e (page

245) are sometimes given. The dose of $B_{12}$ is sometimes escalated to as much as 10,000ug of injection every night. I do recommend the Hydroxocobalamin or the Methylcobolamine. The Cyanocobolamine that is usually given could cause cyanide toxicity in very large doses. The compounding pharmacist will come to your aid and compound the desired B12 preparation so that only 1 or 2cc are needed one dose of 10,000 ug.

The oral cavity frequently needs to be cleaned up with root canal cavitations repaired and the amalgam removed. Staying away from much of the toxins like in regular toothpaste such as fluoride and sodium lauryl sulfate is healthful. Avoiding environmental toxins found in household cleaners and industry is also helpful. One would consider getting rid of the natural toxins in our gastrointestinal tract with the use of colostrum, glutamine, CMO, olive leave extract, probiotic with fructo-oligosaccharide and much natural roughage. See Table 6-II for further therapies. When treatment is given, sometimes there is an accentuation of the disease when toxins get out of the tissues. This lasts for several days to several weeks. It is particularly prominent when one uses MSM, vitamin $B_{12}$ and guaifenesin either together or separately. Other treatments particularly useful in Phase III is that of growth hormone injections, and if available, fetal bovine growth factors. These come from the liver, the thymus, the adrenal, the brain and the mesenchyme.

## $B_{12}$ to the Rescue

Although not as well documented by the orthodox medical community as I would like, vitamin B12 deficiency may be responsible for a small fraction of F Syndrome patients as well as pseudo Alzheimer's Syndrome. A low spinal fluid B12 level has been discovered in some patients with the syndrome. Also a B12 deficiency causes a reversible type of Alzheimer's disease in older patients. Dr. L. Kuwait did a series of patients with spinal spinal puncture fluid and treated with $B_{12}$ injections those who had a low level of spinal fluid $B_{12}$, with a wonderful response. There is no need to do a spinal tap to decide to give a B12 injection. At times I do a serum $B_{12}$ level or its surrogate, a homocystine level. The $B_{12}$ level poorly reflects the tissue level so it is much easier to just give the vitamin. Since $B_{12}$ is poorly absorbed from the intestinal tract, I do give it orally in very high doses, 1000 to 5000 micrograms a day. It is slightly better absorbed when taken under the tongue, but it is best to give 1000 micrograms subcutaneously as a therapeutic trial. Many patients who do have this as their cause of this subset of the syndrome tell me that within one hour, they feel much better. Unfortunately, half of these folks, over the next two months, get down to where they were before, but the other half are cured! I try to have patients inject their $B_{12}$ at home. They start at 1000 ug a week and gradually increase at nights (seems to work better when given just prior to bedtime). When I need higher doses of this, I call in a compounding pharmacy to make *hydroxy*cobalamine or *methyl*cobalamine in concentration as high as 50,000 micrograms per cc. Although more in theory than fact, I do not want to give high doses of *cyano*cobalamine to avoid cyanamide toxicity. Undoubtedly, a placebo affect does occur, but is sorted out in time. A $B_{12}$/taurine combination injection is occasionally advised.

### The E-Dennis Wilson's Syndrome

Another specific entity that can be separated from this F basket of diseases that we call CFS /FM is the E-Dennis Wilson Syndrome. Dr. Wilson discovered, fifteen years ago that, due to physical or emotional trauma, the actual Thyroid hormone that is known as triiodo thyroxin (T3), is not converted from its less active precursor, thyroxin (T4). Hence, the individual has the subtle symptoms and signs of low thyroid (Hypothyroidism). However, compared to the true Hypothyroidism that the medical profession knows, and which is documented by blood tests (a high TSH and a low T4), these poor folks have a normal blood study since their problem is not that they have a low T4, but a low T3! It is the T4, that causes the pituitary in a feedback loop, to produce more or less TSH, but this is not the case with this sub population of patients with low T3 and normal T4.

Dr. Wilson, in his articles and book, details, if there is not enough of the thermogenic T3, the temperature of the body is slightly low. With a lower temperature, the body's enzymes do not function normally and the patient has a host of symptoms, compatible with the F Syndrome. To determine if a patient has this syndrome, he suggests taking ones temperature every three hours, three times a day for three days, with a glass thermometer, orally starting three hours after awakening. The farther the temperature is under 98.6 degrees Fahrenheit, the more likely it is that the patient has this T3 deficiency, the E Dennis Wilson Syndrome.

A therapeutic trial will "prove" in less than two weeks that a low thyroid is the cause of these people's symptoms. Dr. Wilson recommends a low starting dose of long acting T3, 7.5 mg every 12 hours. Then, this is gradually increased until the individual's temperature is "captured", that is to say, when the temperature returns to the average normal of 98.6 degrees Fahrenheit. Most patients will feel concommitently much better at this time. Long acting T3 is made in various doses by a compounding pharmacist and is gradually lowered and then stopped with the patient maintaining their normal T4-T3 conversion and, of course, the patient felling normal.

### Sleep

Not only does nonrestorative sleep occur in the F Syndrome, but so does sleep apnea. I frequently use herbal preparation and melatonin in the evening and bright light in the morning. Obstructive Sleep Apnea, which occurs in 5 percent of men and 3 percent of women, is still another cause of the F Word. This is a collapsing of the upper airways while sleeping. Snorers have a predilection to this abnormality. Although not recognized by the individual, the bed partner, if asked, will make the diagnosis. Sleep fragmentation creates not only fatigue, but also chronic daytime sleepiness. A sleep study referred to as a polysomagram does confirms the disease. This malady is corrected with a nighttime breathing device such as a nose ring adhesive strip above the nose, mouth prosthesis, and a C-Pap (continuous positive airway pressure), and rarely a surgical procedure, opening up the airways by electrical ablation of the excess tissues in the nasal pharyngeal airway.

## Adrenal Fatigue

One more diagnosis to be brought to the surface in this wastebasket of diseases is Subclinical Adrenal Insufficiency or Adrenal Exhaustion. The prominent symptoms in many of these folks, besides fatigue, is light-headedness upon attaining an upright position, termed medically NMH (neuro mediated hypotension). As discussed earlier, hydrocortisone in *small* doses, or the more obtainable and very inexpensive and at the recommended dose very safe Prednisone, is used. A 5 mg pill, in the morning and 2.5 mg (1/2 pill) at noon, greatly improves these patients' symptoms. A physician may do a special test, called a tilt table examination, but it is much easier, and far cheaper to, again, give a two-week therapeutic trial to see if there is a positive response and, hence, not only come up with the correct diagnosis, but the right treatment. My sense, now, is that this is uncommon and feeling better might be only transient. This should be used in conjunction with the ultimate protocol and the judicious use of the drugs and supplements listed in Tables 6-II and III..

## Every Third Day Therapy

The ultimate treatment based not on the usual circadian rhythm that most normals have but the vicious negative consequence cycle of the chronic fatigue. When other therapies have failed, listening to our bodies and acting accordingly will enable us to get through life the best we can although we would all like to do better. We must know our enemy before we can defeat him. There is much scientific literature that can be given such as negative feedback of the Hypophyseal Adrenal axis, the bioactivity of the enzyme 11 beta-hydroxysteroid dexydrogenase (11 beta HSD), the paradoxical hormonal action, free radicals, or given set of down regulated receptors, etc., but this treatment is based on empiricism. Captain David Williams *(davidwms@interpoint.net)* has been expounding on this for months on what he calls ETD (Every Third Day) Therapy, in which the various component of each day is varied to *that* individual and the determination internally (how the body is functioning) and externally (what they need to do). Both Klonopin and the Hydrocortisone (Prednisone) will need a prescription from your cooperative doctor. At times Trazadone or Serozone™ in a low dose can be used instead of Klonopin. These are safe drugs when used as detailed. The basis of this therapy is cortisone, which as mentioned before could be dangerous. Either the more expensive and harder to find Hydrocortisone 25 to 50 mg or the dirt-cheap Prednisone 5 to 7.5 mg is taken in the morning, that we will call day one. If one needs a little boost, if the day is more demanding or if one is not up to their desired self, a repeat *half* dose is again taken in afternoon. Day one should be the day you feel the best and lots of activity should be planned that day, both at home or at work. This also should be the day that much physical exercise be done. Every evening, 1 to 2 mg of Klonopin is taken. This increases the GABA receptors to get a restorative sleep. Day two should still feel pretty good since the Cortisol (Hydrocortisone, Prednisone steroid) is in a limited amount, still in the tissue. Take in the a.m., for women 200 mg of Progesterone, a lot of grapefruit and juice, or real licorice throughout the day. Grapefruit juice can be substituted by grapefruit or even Fresca. Glycyrrhic acid can be used instead of licorice. If one feels nervous, Klonopin 0.5 to 1 mg can be taken to replete the GABA receptors and the "nerves." Again, plan to be active that day and do what needs to be done if one has the time and the energy left, do physical exercise. The evening of day two, take the dose of Klonopin needed to get a good night's sleep. On day three, do *not* take the licorice (glycerrhic acid) or grapefruit juice, but you can take the Klonopin if needed for nerves. Since day three is a day of relaxation, avoid physical activity and stress as much as possible. Depending on your life schedule, you can either do day four like the third day and relax, or if you need to really "hit it" and do the prednisone. Here one can plan their work and play and play and work this plan. Supplements such as Glutamine (see page 227) can be taken anytime of the day for a pick me up.

Once or twice a week two to three buffered aspirin can be taken when one is really down. The other suggestions made earlier in this chapter can be added as needed. Please refer to Tables 6-II and III for supplements and prescription drugs to use judiciously.

Diet is most important. See Chapter Three for details. Specifically, eating for one's blood type, eliminating food allergies (ALCAT) and minimizing wheat, milk, and refined sugars will go a long way to help the "F" word. A full complement of vitamins and minerals are needed. A medical food such as UltraInflamX™, is designed as a low-allergy, rice-based product. This is the following components: antioxidant vitamins and minerals to reduce free-radical generation; phytonutrients, such as rosemary and limonene; sodium sulfate, to support detoxification processes; anti-inflammatory phytonutrients, such as curcumin, to nutritionally support inflammation symptoms; and enhanced levels of vitamins and minerals, such as vitamin C, vitamin $B_3$, zinc, which promote balance in production of pro- and anti-inflammatory cytokines and prostaglandins.

You'll need lots of luck if you have the F Syndrome. A patient, who is assertive and, at times, aggressive, and *knows* his or her disease, will do lots better than a passive one. Remember that I, like all physicians, am human, have clay feet, and do make mistakes and need to be guided by the individual so that we can both journey down the path to the patient's and doctor's enlightenment of this most frustrating disease. In the year 2010 we may know, but in 2001 I give my best educated advice based on both the art and the science of medicine.

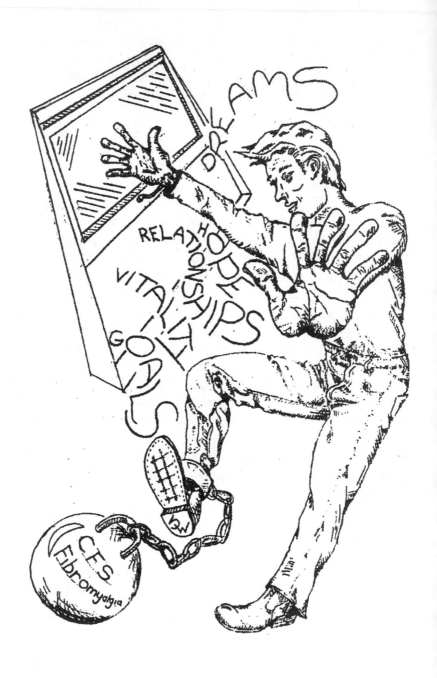

A cartoon given to me by a patient with CFS/FM.

# SEVEN

# Make No Bones About It

Osteoporosis is a silent disease until it announces itself with a sudden fracture or a significant pain and is characterized by a progressive decrease in the density of bones that makes them fragile. In the past, we thought this was only a disease of women. Now we know that twenty-five percent of men are also likely to have this problem, too.

Bones contain minerals like calcium, magnesium, and phosphorus, which make them hard and protein such as collagen that give them good strength. The former is seen as mineral content and correlates positively with bone mineral density and the latter, which includes bone turnover, uses urinary pyridinoline, or N/C telopeptide tests and MRI is at least as important. To maintain bone density, the body requires an adequate supply of calcium and other minerals, and must produce the proper amounts of several hormones; parathyroid hormone, growth hormone, calcitonin, DHEA, estrogen in women, and testosterone in men and women. Also, an adequate supply of vitamin K and D is needed to absorb calcium from food and incorporate it into bones. Bones progressively increase in density until a maximum density is reached, around age 30. After that, bones slowly decrease or deteriorate. If the body isn't able to regulate the mineral content or matrix quality of bones, they become less dense and more fragile, resulting in osteopenia, or in more severe cases, osteoporosis.

Risk factors for disease include systolic hypertension (the top number), taller individuals with generally longer neck of the hip bones, family members both mother and/or father with osteoporosis, insufficient calcium intake, age, chronic lung disease, sedentary lifestyle, White or Oriental race, thin build, no pregnancies, use of certain drugs such as Coumadin® (Warfarin), Dilantin®, corticosteroids and excessive amounts of thyroid hormone. Both coffee and soda pop can cause osteoporosis. The decaffeinated or regular does have a chemical that causes a decrease of bone density. Pop, because of the carbonation, an acid, eats away at the bone. To add insult to injury, the phosphate in the colas play havoc with the calcium in the bone. Also early menopause, cigarette smoking, excessive alcohol consumption, not taking vitamins or hormones from age 45 on, premature graying of the hair, growing up in the Northern latitudes (greater than 40 degrees north and south) and being too thin *(JAMA 14 Feb 2001)* are risk factors. Sudden falling is usually the acute cause of disability. This may be due to a generalized lack of exercise, balance and gait disorders, visual impairment, strokes, certain heart conditions as well as sleeping and/or relaxing pills.

Until recently, I've encouraged my patients to drink milk. We now know that the milk protein, casein, promotes rather than retards osteoporosis. Whey, another protein, is not detrimental. Diane Feskanich in the *American Journal of Epidemiology*, Volume 143, No. 5, tracked medical histories of 78,000 middle-aged women for over ten years and found out women who drank the most milk a day were far more likely to have a broken hip or arm than those who drank less than one glass a week!! That is why the more dairy food people eat, the more likely they are to suffer fractures from osteoporosis. How could anything as wholesome as milk make bones weaker? The answer lies in the fact that the body breaks proteins into its amino acids. It then uses the acids to build muscle and other tissues. An excess of these acids remain in the blood stream, a condition that the body tries to correct. It reaches for the calcium in the bone to neutralize the acid, hence making the bone less dense. Frederick J. Simoons of the University of California at Davis, suggests that it was only because of a genetic aberration that milk became a food staple in northern Europe and North America. Nature normally programs the young for weaning before they reach adulthood by turning down production in early childhood of the enzyme that break down lactose. But a gene mutation inherited by people of northern European descent prevents the production of this enzyme from being turned down as we get older like the rest of the world. What's good for baby calves isn't necessarily good for baby humans or adults. In Asia, where many people drink no milk whatsoever, breast cancer tends to be rare. A prospective study have linked dietary intake of lactose with an increased risk of a subtype of ovarian cancer. According to Harvard's Kathleen Fairfield, MD, women who consumed one or more servings of skim or low-fat milk daily had sixty-six percent higher risk of serous ovarian cancer. For each eleven grams a day increase in lactose consumption (the approximate amount in a glass of milk), the risk of this cancer increased by nineteen percent. Galactose is a metabolite of lactose, and diets high in galactose have been shown to cause abnormal ovaries in mice. Other studies suggest milk causes oocyte depletion and induces ovarian cancer. In India, where people eat more dairy in the form of yogurt, other researchers have documented higher rates of breast cancer. Two areas with higher milk consumption, Scandinavia and the Netherlands, also had higher breast cancer rates. To improve calcium intake and to prevent osteoporosis, in the U.S., dairy products are advised so the solution is the problem. Worldwide, men seem far more likely to die of prostate cancer in countries where dairy consumption is high than in countries where it is low. In the Physicians' Health Study, researchers tracked 20,885 male doctors over 10 years. Those who consumed at least two and a half servings of dairy food per day were thirty percent more likely to develop prostate cancer than doctors who consumed less than half a serving. In other research, the Health Professionals Follow-Up Study had found that men who consumed a large amount of dairy products had a seventy percent higher risk of prostate cancer.

Paradoxically, in older people the problem seems not to

be the calcium as much as not having as much protein, which is reflected by their serum albumin, and is normally assessed in most physician's offices. For a variety of reasons (poor dentition, decreased stomach hydrochloric acid, reduction of digestive enzymes, living alone, etc.) older people have poor nutrition. Additional calcium intake has benefits in preventing heart disease, particularly by the reduction in blood pressure, colon cancer, premenstrual syndrome and kidney stones. To prevent stones, it is usually recommended the calcium be taken with meals. Bone density decreases slowly, especially in people who have older age mild disease called osteopenia. At first, there are no symptoms. Osteopenia proceeds into osteoporosis. When bone density decreases so much that bones collapse or break, aching bone pain and deformities develop. Chronic back pain may occur if vertebrae collapse (vertebral crush fractures). The weakened vertebrae may collapse spontaneously or after a slight injury. Usually, severe pain starts suddenly in the back and worsens when a person stands or walks. The area may be sore when touched, but usually the soreness goes away gradually after a few weeks or months. If several vertebrae break, an abnormal curvature of the spine (a dowager's hump) may develop, causing additional muscle strain and soreness as well as abdominal protuberance.

Other bones may fracture, often because of minor stress or as noted above, a fall. One of the most serious fractures is a hip fracture, a major cause of disability and loss of independence in the elderly. Many patients enter the hospital and never come out the same. Although there are far fewer hip fractures in men than in women (81,000 versus 271,000 in 1998), the mortality rate for men in the year following hip fracture is twice than in women. Fracture of the arm bone (radius) where it joins the wrist, called a Colles' fracture, is also common. In addition, fractures tend to heal slowly in people who have osteoporosis and are more painful.

In people who have a fracture, the diagnosis of osteoporosis is based on a combination of symptoms, physical examination and special bone "x-rays." Further testing may be needed to rule out treatable conditions that might lead to osteoporosis. However, osteoporosis can be diagnosed before a fracture occurs. Several tests that assess bone density can help with the diagnosis. We use a DEXA (Dual Energy X-ray Absorptiometry) of the hand taking just two minutes to perform. It correlates well with the more expensive studies. The better diagnosis of this bone disease is an MRI of the hip, wrist, vertebra and heel. Bone biopsy with microscopic and MRI is the best method, but because of it being invasive, it is used only for research. Today, we make the diagnosis using a DEXA, which give both a T and a Z score. The T score is the one clinicians commonly use, although there is also a Z score. This is the patients comparison with other people of the same age. Since we should strive physically to be as young as we can, the Z score will soon be discarded. If the density value is more than 1 standard deviation below a young healthy normal average (T-Score), there is *osteopenia*, or if greater than 2.5 there is *osteoporosis*. Each standard deviation, which represents a ten percent reduction of bone mineral density, doubles the fracture risk! There is an accentuated direct correlation of the score improvement and a decreased risk of fracture. For example, an eight percent increase in BMD improves the reduction of risk for a fracture by fifty percent! This demonstrates the value of three-dimensional protein matrix improvement as well as the mineralization of the bone.

Preventing osteopenia and osteoporosis is more successful than treating it. Prevention involves maintaining or increasing bone density by consuming an adequate amount of calcium and magnesium, engaging in weight-bearing exercise and for some people, taking natural products. Vitamin $B_6$, C, D, folic acid, the minerals magnesium (500mg), strontium (50mg), silica (20mg), zinc (30mg), copper (3mg), and boron (1-3mg) are recommended. Cutting ones salt intake in half enables the body to retain up to 20% more calcium.

From teenagers on, consider increasing our calcium and magnesium. Vitamin D is found in vitamin supplements or with mild sun exposure (please don't get burned). However, most folks who are trying to prevent osteoporosis take calcium and magnesium in tablet form, but it is far better to eat an over-abundance of vegetables such as kale, spinach, broccoli, beans and sea vegetables. Please see Table 7-I. Other sources of natural calcium are sardines, tofu and calcium fortified orange or grapefruit juice. The latter has more calcium than a glass of milk and has Fruit-Cal®, which is mostly calcium citrate, the most easily absorbed calcium produced. In a study published in JAMA Vol. 284, No.11 in September 2000, many calcium formulations contain lead and thereby may be a health concern.

If you must take inorganic calcium, many different preparations are available. Some include supplemental vitamin D. About 1.5 grams of calcium each day is recommended. It is best to take the calcium with meals and with 500mg of vitamin C. Magnesium 200 to 400mg a day also helps to make and keep strong bones. When osteopenia is diagnosed, calcium, magnesium and boron are recommended. Although I do not necessarily advocate it, beer may be good for the bone. The hops in beer contain three chemicals that stop the breakdown of the bone. Tea, both green and black, according to an English study published in *American Journal of Clinical Nutrition* (2000; 71, 1003-7) protected against osteoporosis in older women.

Weight-bearing exercise, such as walking and stair-climbing, also increases bone density. Bones need an essential tensile/torque force to stimulate strengthening mineral protein complex.Exercises that don't involve essential weight bearing, such as swimming, don't seem to increase bone density. Tai Chi and yoga is very helpful in that it is not only a strain/twisting weight bearing exercise, but enhances balance that tends to prevent falls. Because estrogen helps maintain bone density in women, some women take estrogen, sometimes with progesterone and androgen after menopause. These hormone supplements are given in doses that simulate the protective hormonal balance found in menstruating younger women. Estrogen replacement therapy is most effective when started in the perimenopausal years, but studies have shown that starting it later can still slow bone loss and reduce the risk of fractures. Testosterone replacement is frequently given to women and even more so to men for treatment and protection of osteoporosis.

Postmenopausal women may be given hormone replacement in the form of estrogen or Evista® , an estrogen-like drug. Evista may actually prevent breast cancer. Although there may be a slight tendency for estrogen to cause breast cancer, one needs to consider that almost three times as many women a day die of a fractured hip compared to breast cancer!! Men are placed on testosterone. Now there is an easy to use prescription gel, which is far better than the patches and injections given previously. Both the gel and the patches are expensive compared to the once or twice monthly injections. Vitamin D in large amounts, such as 50,000 units (a prescription), which is inexpensive, is taken once a week usually on Sunday. Another vitamin which has recently surfaced in prevention and treatment of osteoporosis is vitamin K, either naturally in the green leafy vegetables or in a pill of 1 to 10 mg daily (see pages 161-164). Taking Hydrochlorothiazide, a diuretic, in a small dose (12.5 mg) daily is dirt cheap and extremely effective according to the research published in the *Annals of Int. Med.*, Oct. 5, 2000. In more severe cases, oral 30mg Actonel® or 70mg Fosamax® given weekly, nasal Miacalcin® used daily, possibly Statin cholesterol lowering drugs, long-acting fluoride, injectable synthetic parathormone, Forteo® *(New Eng. Journal of Med.,* May 10, 2001), and the injectable Human Growth Hormone, are prescribed by physicians. In refractory cases, several or all can be given to the patient.

Fractures resulting from osteoporosis must be treated. For hip fractures, usually part or all of the hip is replaced. A wrist fracture is placed in a cast or reset surgically. When vertebrae collapse and cause excruciating back pain, supportive back braces, analgesics and physical therapy are used, but the pain tends to last three to four months. Recently several surgical procedures have been shown to locally strengthen the bone. The orthopedic glue methylmethacrylate can be injected into the crushed vertebrae giving it support, preventing the deformity and subsequently relieving the pain. Because of the pain, there is a higher incidence of suicide in these poor folks. Although traditionally not thought of as a silent killer it is. As many as 300,000 cases a year of women with hip fractures in the U.S. alone occur with a fair proportion of deaths. Most importantly, the patient needs to be started on an intensive bone building program as outlined above. The use of Miacalcin may particularly helpful in that it not only improves the osteoporosis, but decreases the bone pain significantly.

. **Table 7-I**

## BONE FOOD

| Food | Serving Size | Calcium Content (mg) |
|---|---|---|
| **Dairy products** | | |
| Milk (an unhealthy source) | 1 cup | 302 |
| Fat-free Yogurt | 8 oz | 100-400 |
| with added milk solids | | |
| American cheese | 1 oz | 172 |
| Swiss | 1 oz | 272 |
| Ricotta | 1/2 cup | 337 |
| Cottage | 1 cup | 155 |
| | | |
| **Other** | | |
| Broccoli (fresh) | 1 cup | 176 |
| Vegetarian Baked Beans | 1 cup | 128 |
| Collard greens | 1 cup | 150 |
| Kidney Beans (red, boiled) | 1 cup | 116 |
| Sardines | 3 oz | 373 |
| Grapefruit juice (calcium fortified) | 1 cup | 402 |
| Orange juice (calcium fortified) | 1 cup | 300 |
| Dried figs | 10 | 270 |
| Tofu (raw) | 1/2 cup | 260 |

# UNDERSTANDING BONE DENSITY REPORTS

The usual dual energy bone densitometry (DEXA) scan is two-dimensional. It measures the mineral content of the bone and divides by the surface area to determine "bone mineral density" (BMD) in $mg/cm^2$. This is compared to a standard database and reported as T or Z scores.

## T and Z scores

The reported Z score is the measurement compared with a database matched for age, gender and race. Statistically a Z score is the number of standard deviations (SD) from the mean, a positive number is above the mean, a negative score below it. With some systems, it is adjusted for body weight as well. For the "T score" or "Young Z score," the bone density is compared with peak bone density, that for an average 30-year-old. The T scores are specific for the type of machine and the database used by the manufacturer.

## Diagnostic criteria

The majority of hip fractures occur in people with a bone mineral density 2.5 SD below the mean peak bone density (a T score of -2.5 or worse).

Peripheral bone densitometry is useful for screening but the WHO diagnostic criteria are based on central (spine and hip) DEXA scans in postmenopausal women. The diagnostic criteria are:

BMD decreased ≥1 SD    osteopenia
                ≥2 SD    osteoporosis
                              (National Osteoporosis Foundation)
              ≥2.5 SD    osteoporosis
                              (World Health Organization)
          with fracture    severe osteoporosis

Each standard deviation is about a 10% change in BMD and about doubles fracture risk. These criteria are for labeling and billing purposes and do not determine who should or should not be treated. Anyone with decreased bone density is either a candidate for therapy or, at least, prevention of further loss.

## What if the scores differ for different bones?

It is not unusual to have different densities in different bones. In the spine, the posterior elements constitute about 50% of the mineral content. Osteoarthritis of the spine and, to a lesser extent, aortic calcification can increase the measured density. Collapsed vertebrae or marked spinal deformity can invalidate the spinal measurement. Generally, therapeutic decisions are based on the lowest reading. T is for The Primary and Z is for Zecondary, and a Z score that is -1.5 or worse indicates that the bone density is well below age-matched peers and suggests that there may be another (secondary) cause for the osteopenia. The most common causes are hormonal, medications, and low calcium, magnesium, vitamin D and K intake. These can be caused in addition to poor intake by decreased absorption or excessive loss. Primary osteoporosis is the term used when another cause is not determined and is reflected in a low T score.

Hypogonadism is a major cause of bone loss, not only in postmenopausal women, but also in women who have amenorrhea associated with eating disorders and/or excessive physical activity. Men with hypogonadism also are at high risk for osteopenia.

One of the most common causes of bone loss is prolonged cortisone use. These steroids promote teardown of protein and antagonize vitamin D action. Anticonvulsants accelerate breakdown of vitamin D. Patients with a gastrectomy or chronic intestinal disorders may have fat malabsorption and vitamin D deficiency. Prolonged hyperthyroidism, frequently by taking thyroid hormone, has been associated with decreased bone density. An overactive parathyroid gland is another secondary cause.

## ADDITIONAL TESTING

The clinical picture will determine what other tests are indicated (see below). Blood levels of 25-hydroxy-vitamin D will reflect body stores of vitamin D. A low 24-hour urinary calcium excretion also can confirm low calcium absorption and/or intake.

**Biochemical Markers of Bone Turnover**

High levels of urinary N-telopeptides, or other markers for breakdown products of Type 1 collagen, may be associated with an increased risk for fractures. However, currently available blood or urinary tests for biochemical markers of bone formation or loss are not reproducible enough for use in screening. They may be useful in showing the effect of therapy; changes in biochemical parameters can occur long before an increase in bone density can be seen.

Markers of bone formation, such as osteocalcin or bone-specific alkaline phosphatase, are rarely measured except in specialized research centers.

**Calcium and/or Vitamin D metabolism**

Serum calcium, phosphorus, alkaline phosphatase (all should be normal in osteoporosis)

25-hydroxy-vitamin D

24-hour urinary calcium and creatinine

Intact parathyroid hormone (PTH) if hypercalcemic or hypocalcemic

**Gonadal function:** Testosterone, FSH, LH, estradiol

**Other: General Health**

Blood count, metabolic profiles, TSH (thyroid)

Protein electrophoresis for multiple myeloma

*There is more than sticks and stones to break the bones.*

# Figure 7-I.
## Osteoporosis

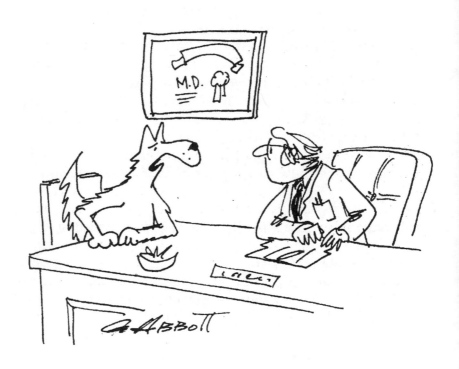

*"Doctor, what can I do to prevent bone loss?"*

**EIGHT**

# A Pause Not to Take

"No doubt about it," hormonal replacement benefits outweigh the risks. Unfortunately, too many women in our country are not taking hormones because of the false concern that they may cause cancer. Today, a woman who is age 50 and in good health, could very well spend half her lifetime in a postmenopausal hormone imbalance and hence, subject to increase of morbid problems mentioned later. This is the only endocrinopathy (hormone abnormality) in all of medicine that is not routinely replaced. Certainly, if the patient has a low thyroid level, doctors prescribe thyroid. If she has low adrenal output, we give her cortisone. No physician would dare withhold insulin from a diabetic, but most physicians are not giving female hormones to those who need it most. Recent statistics show that less than 30% of postmenopausal women receive hormonal replacement and that 50% of women that were prescribed this, discontinue their medicine within one year. There are two cancers that may be related to hormone replacement. One is uterine (endometrial) and the other is breast.

Researchers unequivocally has shown that women who take unopposed estrogen, (that is estrogen without progesterone), there is a four fold risk of endometrial (uterine) cancer. However, this is a very slow growing cancer commonly picked up because of postmenopausal bleeding and is rarely, if ever fatal under these circumstances. However, if she does take progesterone along with estrogen, the inci-

of endometrial cancer is even less than if she were taking any hormone. Regarding breast cancer, statistically one in nine women will develop this. These figures are only correct if the patient lives to be 105. In a women who is in good health at age 50 and has not had breast cancer, her risk of dying from breast cancer is only 2%. This means 98% of the time, she's going to die of something else other than breast cancer!!! This something else is usually cardiovascular disease like a stroke, which could be a fate worse than cancer. However, many women are blind-sided by their false impression of hormones causing their breast cancer.

In a study in JAMA 2000 (Volume 283, Number 4), by Dr. C. Sihair involving 46,000 women followed for fifteen years, there was a slight increase in breast cancer if the woman took both estrogen and progesterone. However, most of these women took a *synthetic* progesterone and were *cycled* monthly. This is another reason to take natural hormones and to take them daily rather than sequentially.

Today, with mammography we're catching breast cancer earlier and earlier. Patients will have a 95% chance of long term survival, even if she does have breast cancer. There are other factors that cause breast cancer which many women do not consider. If she waits until she is 30 years old to have her first child rather than having her first child in her 20's, her risk of breast cancer increased 50%. If she is a little on the heavy side, her risk goes up another 50%. If she drinks, smokes, or eats too much fat, the risk of breast cancer goes up another 20%. On the other hand, if she decides to take hormone replacement and has been on it for five years, her cancer risk may go up less than 5%. A recent study shows she may have even less of a chance of an aggressive cancer. A review article in *The New England Journal of* Medicine (October 12, 2000) indicates hormone replacement impairs both the sensitivity and specificity of a mammogram in diagnosing breast cancer or recurrence of such. Stopping the hormones for two weeks before the procedure restores the accuracy of the study. Also, having a timely period once a year may be good for the woman. Quadrant biopsies with fine needles are becoming more popular in women who have abnormal calcification on their mammogram. This prevents the surgery and scarring of the breast and is very accurate.

The advantages of taking female hormones are great. Gynecological problems such as vaginal dryness, painful intercourse, decreased libido, vaginal infections, leakage of urine and recurrent bladder infections are markedly improved. The uncomfortable symptoms like hot flashes, night sweats, mood and sleep disturbances improve within 48 hours of taking female hormones. As noted above, the prevention of cardiovascular disease, in particular, a heart attack and stroke is markedly prevented by hormonal replacement. Osteopenia, or its big bad brother, osteoporosis can cause pain in mild cases and fractures in severe cases in women not taking female hormones as noted in Chapter Seven. Moreover, hormone replacement improves memory and decreases brain cell loss in Alzheimer's disease. Cancer of the colon, caries of teeth, decreased vision due to cataracts and macular degeneration occur more often in women who do not take hormones. Although not nearly as important to physicians, but very important to the individual, premature aging of the person occurs more in women who chose not to take female hormones. Wrinkling of the skin, decreased vibrancy of the hair, slow growing and cracking of the nails are common signs of estrogen deficiency.

Natural hormones have been shown to be safer than the synthetic. At this time, I recommend a combination of what the ovaries used to make in the form of estriol ($E_3$) and estradiol ($E_2$). I usually prescribe these in the exact ratio the ovaries made in the past. There is another natural hormone, estrone ($E_1$) that has been implicated more in breast cancer. I do not therefore add this to the regime. Additionally, the ovary did make progesterone and a small amount of androgens. This androgen is essential to normal sexual desire. It helps promote weight loss, improves the integrity of muscle and bone and exercise tolerance. I recommend taking the combination hormone every day of the year. By six months, there is no more bleeding and the monthly "visit" that plagued a lady during her youth no longer occurs in her maturity.

"One size doesn't fit all." I give what is usual for the average woman; that is 2.5mg estrogen, 100mg progesterone and 1mg of testosterone. Depending on the patient's experience with this mixture, various components are increased or decreased until she is not only free of symptoms, but her body functions as it did when she was younger. Should the breasts become tender, we reduce the estrogen. Should she have fluid retention, mood swings and/or migraine headaches, we decrease the estrogen or increase the progesterone. On the other hand, if there were to be excess hair growth we would decrease the androgen. If the uterus is still present, there is always a chance for breakthrough bleeding and if one stops the estrogen suddenly there is a good chance for a heavy period. There are blood tests available that will show not only how effective hormone replacement therapy is in preventing problems in the future (FSH/LH levels) and also a test (Estradiol) to determine if one will have breakthrough bleeding with treatment and when stopping a very heavy period. This test is easily performed in the lab along with the FSH/LH levels, frequently done the same day the blood is drawn. A Dutch researcher (vandWeijer) in *The Journal of Obstetrics and Gynecology* (April 1999) revealed that if the serum Estradiol level before treatment is greater than 49 (pg/ml), the chances of bleeding were significant compared to if the level is less than this. Therefore, by doing Estradiol, FSH/LH levels, in which cases the latter should be less than 20 indicates the correct hormone dose. In the past, doctors would just give what they felt was the proper dose, but now we are more scientific with the lab studies in combination with a woman's symptoms if too much or too little hormone. A recent book (Your Hormone Type by Dr. Collins) gives a questionnaire to help me decide what starting dose of the estrogen, progesterone, and androgen is needed. It also gives many non-prescriptive alternatives to hormone replacement.

There are other ways to go other than taking hormones and much of this is mentioned in Dr. Collins' book. Black cohash for hot flashes, chaste berry for mood symptoms, ginkgo biloba for memory and reversing senility, ginseng to improve sexual function, passion flower to overcome insomnia, valerian to help one sleep and the various soy products that will function as estrogens to some extent are detailed. Soy does contain isoflavones, particularly Genistein and Diazosin. Phytoestrogens (plant source estrogen-like compounds which are diphenolic compounds) are converted into estrogen-like substances in the gastrointestinal tract. More importantly, phytoestrogens prevent the xenoestrogens (foreign and toxic estrogen) from adhering to the estrogen receptor. It is the xenoestrogens which are thought to stimulate cells to produce abnormally and in some cases, even to the cause of cancer. Natural and phytoestrogens will diminish this by protecting the receptor site from these noxious agents. Xenoestrogens are caused by contamination of pesticides, other hydrocarbons, and chemicals in our air, water, food and on the skin. In our modern society it is most difficult to eliminate these from our environment.

There may be enough evidence to support the use of phytoestrogens to prevent breast cancer and there are almost conclusive studies that at least soy protein prevents cardiovascular disease by lowering LDL cholesterol and triglycerides, raising the good HDL cholesterol and causing a dilation rather than constriction in an atherosclerotic vessel. Also, it has been shown that there was a correlation to an improved estrogenic vaginal cytology. However, the research in soy is still under development.

The hormones should be given in the perimenopausal period before women actually start menopause. A woman in her mid-forties who is having late periods, slight hot flashes, an increase in mood swings, a new sleep disorder and a family history of early menopause would indicate the need to start hormone treatment soon, rather than waiting for the full blown menopause. Studies show much less bone loss, an earlier improvement in lipids and even a lesser incidence of Alzheimers if the hormones are started while the young lady is still having periods. However, better late than never and I do start an 80-year-old woman on hormones so that she can have a longer and a better life.

# Lydia Pinkham's Compound: The Recipe

Patented 1875

Black cohosh
(cimicifuga racemosa [L.] Nutt.):
6 ounces
Fenugreek seed
(Trigonella foenum graecum L.):
12 ounces
Life root
(Senecio aureus L.):
6 ounces
Pleurisy root
(Asclepias tuberosa L.):
6 ounces
Unicorn root
(Aletris farinosa L.):
8 ounces
Ethel Alcohol 18%

# NINE

# The Saint of John Hopkins

Born in rural Canada in the 1850s, the greatest clinician in the last two centuries came into being. I mentioned Dr. Herzler in Chapter one, but William Osler has been my medical hero since I entered medical school 40 years ago. From McGill University, he emigrated to America via the University of Pennsylvania, our countries oldest and at that time, the best medical school. He then started a school that within a decade, became America's best and has retained this status even until today, John Hopkins. In 1905 he was awarded the most prestigious medical position in the world, the Regius professorship of medicine in Oxford.

It was he who brought medical students out of the lecture halls, into the wards where bedside teaching was embraced. The clinical clerkship came into being, and practical rather than theoretical teaching emerged. He stated "the best teacher is the patient himself." Although he wrote the most read textbook in the world, *The Principles and Practice of Medicine* (which went through 16 editions, the last being published in 1947, 26 years after his death), he claimed to teach medicine without a book is like sailing in an uncharted sea, but to learn medicine without the patient is like *never* going to sea at all! So then and now, both the patient and the book are needed to produce a physician. The time was right for him to flourish. The decade of the 1880s was perhaps the most exciting brief period that had ever occurred in the 2,300-year history of Western medicine. The germ theory of Louis Pasteur, Robert Koch, and Joseph Lister gained acceptance during that time, and one disease after another was shown to be caused by some specific organism. Medical thinking was transformed. Dr. Osler was in the middle of this catalysis. Because of him and in particular, his textbook, English displaced German, the then language of medicine. William Osler was one of very few men on this planet equipped fully to comprehend the magnitude of the changes about to take place in research and later in practice. His unique expertness with the microscope, his studies with leading scientists in Vienna and Berlin, his focus on the study of pathological tissues as guides to the understanding of disease processes, his youthful energies and enthusiasms were present. All of these combined to guarantee that the new discoveries rapidly found practical use in his hands, not only in the study of sickness but also in the teaching of students.

In 1884 the medical school of the University of Pennsylvania, where Ben Franklin had been, called Osler to the chair of medicine. Osler's departure was a devastating blow to McGill. Their finest teacher was escorted to the train station by almost the entire student body. He was on his way to the next phase of the journey that would lead inevitably to Baltimore. The geographic progression southward was partnered with the academic progression upward. In Philadelphia, Osler gave free rein to his determination that autopsy and microscopic study were the keys to understanding the evolution of disease. Osler had said that he "wished he could be present, having taken such a lifelong interest in the his own medical history. Indeed his own autopsy was performed in his home, and course he was there but not as the physician.

Even in the flood of new scientific information he was discovering, however, Osler never neglected the humanity of his patients. The medical statistics and massing of cases into groups that were necessary to elucidate clinical conditions did not mislead him into forgetting the distinctiveness of each person who came under his care. I tried to emulate him in his approach to the patient and teaching, but an Osler

I will never be. It is true that I did a fair job of teaching and was very successful in the practice of medicine. New discoveries in medicine are progressing at an even faster pace than in the late 1800s, but my personality and perhaps my IQ being less than Osler's has held me back. Despite this, I do try to live up to the word "doctor," which comes form the Latin word "docera," to teach. To teach students and patients alike has become my personal byword for these 40 some years as a physician. Noted in Chapters one and two, a well-informed patient will receive the best of medical care. The combination of Herzler's Horse and Buggy philosophy and Osler's practical approach to technology is what today's medical practice needs today. Importantly, technology should not overcome the humanity of medicine! This was true ten thousand years ago and is today. A responsible physician with a knowledgeable patient is the key to lock in the best health care possible. Hopefully this book has given you some of this perspective.

*It is not how hard one tries, but how well they succeed that counts.*

*— Anonymous*

# THE "NEW" HIPPOCRATIC OATH

## *Patient-Physician Covenant*
### *Tulane University School of Medicine, Class of 2003*

*Medicine is, at its center, a moral enterprise grounded in a covenant of trust. This covenant obliges physicians to be competent and to use their competence in the patient's best interests. Physicians, therefore, are both intellectually and morally obliged to act as advocates for the sick wherever their welfare is threatened and for their health at all times.*

*Today, this covenant of trust is significantly threatened. From within, there is growing legitimization of the physician's materialistic self-interest; from without, for-profit forces press the physician into the role of commercial agent to enhance the profitability of health care organizations. Such distortions of the physician's responsibility degrade the physician-patient relationship that is the central element and structure of clinical care. To capitulate to these alterations of the trust relationship is to significantly alter the physician's role as healer, carer, helper, and advocate for the sick and for the health of all.*

*By its traditions and very nature, medicine is a special kind of human activity—one that cannot be pursued effectively without the virtues of humility, honesty, intellectual integrity, compassion, and effacement of excessive self-interest. These traits mark physicians as members of a moral community dedicated to something other than its own self-interest.*

*Our first obligation must be to serve the good of those persons who seek our help and trust us to provide it. Physicians, as physicians, are not, and must never be, commercial entrepreneurs, gateclosers, or agents of fiscal policy that runs counter to our trust. Any defection from the primacy of the patient's well-being places the patient at risk by treatment that may compromise quality of or access to medical care.*

*We believe the medical profession must reaffirm the primacy of its obligation to the patient through national, state, and local professional societies; our academic, research, and hospital organizations; and especially through personal behavior. As advocates for the promotion of health and support of the sick, we are called upon to discuss, defend, and promulgate medical care by every ethical means available. Only by caring and advocating for the patient can the integrity of our profession be affirmed. Thus we honor our covenant of trust with patients.*

# INDEX

Linoleic Acid 77
Lipids 234
Lipoic Acid 220,231,232
Lithium 176
Llyod, Andrew 267,270
Lovastatin 167,244
Lucidril 221
Luetolin 168
Lupus 42,190,222,225,227
Lutein 233
Lycopene 233,234,235
Macular Degeneration
   114,118,119,120,182,233
Magnesium
   7,176,177,289,262,276,279,293,294
Magnesium Deficiency Syndrome 11
Magnetic Therapy 11
Manganese 177
Mayo Clinic Proceedings 113
Mayo Clinic Diet 93
Mayo Clinic 18
McKenzie, Clancy, M.D. 45
McKenzie, Robin, M.D. 273
Meditation 32
Melatonin 10,235,246
Memo Puretm 239
Mendosa, Rick (Glycemic Index) 86
Menopausal Symptoms 49
Menopause 2
Metabolic Disease 62
Methylation 246
Methylmalonic acid 150
Mevacor® 244
MFS 253
Miacalcin® 296
Migraine 11,50,57,228,254,256,279
Milk 98,290,291,294,296
Milk Thistle 204
Mind-Body Medicine 32
Mitochondrial Theory, The 127
Mitral Valve Prolapse 254,256
Modafinil 213
Modiracetam 240
Molybdenum 178
Monosaturated Fats 72,76
Monoterpenes 94
Movidyn® 209
MSM 181,237,282

Multiple Chemical Senitivity 254,256
Multiple Sclerosis 41,154,279,280
Muscular Dystrophy 169
Mycoplasma 262
Myofascial Syndrome (MFS) 255,261,264
Myricetin 168
N-Acetyl Cysteine (NAC) 227,237
NADH 147
Nathanelsz, Peter, "Life in the Womb" 126
National Institutes of Health 221
Neo-Lidocantonr® 250
Nervonic Acid 77
Neural Arc Theory 264
Neural Therapy 265
Neurocirculatory Asthenia 268
Neuroendocrine Theory 129
Neurokinin-I 260
Neurology 76
Neuropeptide-Y3 60
Neuropeptides 22
Neurosomatic Syndrome 254,255,263
Neuroticism 255
New England Journal of Medicine
   10,72,112,131,267,300
Newland, B. Sherwin, M.D. "Doctors:
   The Biography of Medicine" 1
Newton, Isaac 21
NHIDS 268
Nicetile 212
Nicotinamide 147
NIDS 255
Niehaus, Paul 127
Nieper, Hans 151
Nitroprusside 153
NLEA (Nutritional Labeling
   Educational Act) 65
NMDA 260,261,266
NMH 260,273
Noni Juice 238
Noodis 239
Nootrop 239
Nootropyl 239
NOPE 259
Noradrenaline 257
Normabrain 212,239
Norzetam 239
Novocetam 239
NSAIDs 92,221,246